'The book provides a rich resource for all who are interested in the practice of supervision and in developing their work as supervisors.'

Stephen Crawford, *Psychoanalytic Psychotherapist, Supervisor and Fellow of the Foundation for Psychotherapy and Counselling (FPC). Formerly Senior Programme Manager at WPF Therapy in London.*

'A compendium of all that is essential for anyone taking up the role of supervisor for the first time; experienced supervisors will find, a helpful reference manual that touches on the most significant aspects of the subject.'

Susanna Wright, *Jungian Training and Supervising Analyst. Society of Analytical Psychology (SAP).*

Psychodynamic and Psychoanalytic Supervision

In this comprehensive and informative book, Christine Driver provides a systematic overview of the key issues that a supervisor of psychodynamic and psychoanalytic therapy needs to consider and understand in order to work effectively and dynamically.

Psychodynamic and Psychoanalytic Supervision: A Contemporary Introduction examines key elements of the supervisory role, from container, contract, frames and boundaries to the dynamics of the supervisory relationship, unconscious processes, including the reflection process and parallel process, evaluation and assessment and ethics. Driver considers the importance of learning and exploration for both supervisor and supervisee, and provides guidance on how to effectively conduct these sessions. She provides clinical examples of in person and online supervision and considers learning theory, neuroscience and systemic ideas to support the reader on their own journey. The systematic approach to the key dynamics are outlined to enable readers to generate understanding about the patient and their internal world, as well as the development of the work of the supervisee with their patients.

Part of the Routledge Introductions to Contemporary Psychoanalysis series, this book is a rich resource for all analysts, counsellors and therapists who work psychodynamically or psychoanalytically as supervisors or who are conducting supervision training.

Christine Driver is a Psychoanalytic Psychotherapist and Analytical Psychologist based in London, UK. She is an Honorary Member of the British Association for Psychoanalytic and Psychodynamic Supervision (BAPPS) and has taught, supervised and run supervision trainings. She is the author of *The Self and the Quintessence: A Jungian Perspective* (2020).

Routledge Introductions to Contemporary Psychoanalysis

Series Editor: Aner Govrin
Executive Editor: Yael Peri Herzovich

This comprehensive series illuminates the intricate landscape of psychoanalytic theory and practice. In this collection of concise yet illuminating volumes, we delve into the influential figures, groundbreaking concepts, and transformative theories that shape the contemporary psychoanalytic landscape. At the heart of each volume lies a commitment to clarity, accessibility, and depth. Our expert authors, renowned scholars and practitioners in their respective fields, guide readers through the complexities of psychoanalytic thought with precision and enthusiasm. Whether you are a seasoned psychoanalyst, a student eager to explore the field, or a curious reader seeking insight into the human psyche, our series offers a wealth of knowledge and insight.

Erich Fromm: A Contemporary Introduction
Sandra Buechler

Narcissism: A Contemporary Introduction
Richard Wood

The Death Drive: A Contemporary Introduction
Rossella Valdrè

Depression: A Contemporary Introduction
Marianne Leuzinger-Bohleber

Ronald Fairbairn: A Contemporary Introduction
David P. Celani

For more information about this series, please visit: www.routledge.com/Routledge-Introductions-to-Contemporary-Psychoanalysis/book-series/ICP

Psychodynamic and Psychoanalytic Supervision

A Contemporary Introduction

Christine Driver

Routledge
Taylor & Francis Group

LONDON AND NEW YORK

Designed cover image: © Michal Heiman, Asylum 1855–2020, The Sleeper (video, psychoanalytic sofa and Plate 34), exhibition view, Herzliya Museum of Contemporary Art, 2017.

First published 2026
by Routledge
4 Park Square, Milton Park, Abingdon, Oxon OX14 4RN

and by Routledge
605 Third Avenue, New York, NY 10158

Routledge is an imprint of the Taylor & Francis Group, an informa business

British Library Cataloguing-in-Publication Data
A catalogue record for this book is available from the British Library

ISBN: 978-1-032-80269-5 (hbk)
ISBN: 978-1-032-74700-2 (pbk)
ISBN: 978-1-003-49613-7 (ebk)

DOI: 10.4324/9781003496137

Typeset in Times New Roman
by Taylor & Francis Books

Contents

Figures

Series Editor Preface

Routledge Introductions to Contemporary Psychoanalysis is one of the most prominent psychoanalytic publishing ventures of our day. The series' aim is to become an encyclopedia of psychoanalysis, with each entry given its own book.

This comprehensive series illuminates the intricate landscape of psychoanalytic theory and practice. In this collection of concise yet illuminating volumes, we delve into the influential figures, groundbreaking concepts, and transformative theories that shape the contemporary psychoanalytic landscape.

At the heart of each volume lies a commitment to clarity, accessibility, and depth. Our expert authors, renowned scholars and practitioners in their respective fields, guide readers through the complexities of psychoanalytic thought with precision and enthusiasm. Whether you are a seasoned psychoanalyst, a student eager to explore the field, or a curious reader seeking insight into the human psyche, our series offers a wealth of knowledge and insight.

Each volume serves as a gateway into a specific aspect of psychoanalytic theory and practice. From the pioneering works of Sigmund Freud to the innovative contributions of modern theorists such as Antonino Ferro and Michal Eigen, our series covers a diverse range of topics, including seminal figures, key concepts, and emerging trends. Whether you are interested in classical psychoanalysis, object relations theory, or the intersection of neuroscience and psychoanalysis, you will find a wealth of resources within our collection.

One of the hallmarks of our series is its interdisciplinary approach. While rooted in psychoanalytic theory, our volumes draw upon insights from psychology, philosophy, sociology, and other disciplines to offer a holistic understanding of the human mind and its complexities.

Each volume in the series is crafted with the reader in mind, balancing scholarly rigor with engaging prose. Whether you are embarking on your journey into psychoanalysis or seeking to deepen your understanding of specific topics, our series provides a clear and comprehensive roadmap.

Moreover, our series is committed to fostering dialogue and debate within the psychoanalytic community. Each volume invites readers to critically engage with the material, encouraging reflection, discussion, and further exploration.

We invite you to join us on this journey of discovery as we explore the ever-evolving landscape of psychoanalysis.

Aner Govrin

Preface

I have been training supervisors and writing about supervision since 1990 and so it was a privilege to be asked to write this book. Becoming and being a supervisor is a process in its own right and requires new and additional skills. This book is aimed at those psychoanalytic and psychodynamic professionals who are moving into the supervisory profession or who want to develop their understanding of being a supervisor.

The role of a supervisor has developed considerably since the beginnings of the psychoanalytic and psychotherapy profession as a result of a growing understanding of the complexity of the supervisory relationship in relation to the supervisee, the patient and the unconscious. The roles and tasks of a supervisor in relation to this complexity is the focus of this book.

Beginning with the first step of becoming and being a supervisor the chapters take the reader through the areas that need to be considered when working as a supervisor. Chapter 1 outlines the key areas involved in being a supervisor, either in person or online, and identifies the roles and tasks of a supervisor in relation to the dynamics of the supervisory relationship. Chapter 2 moves on to consider the parameters and dynamics of the supervisory container and Chapter 3 examines the complexities of the supervisory relationship and the supervisory alliance including issues of diversity and difference. Supervision within the psychoanalytic and psychotherapy profession also requires a depth of understanding in relation to the dynamics and impact of the unconscious and Chapter 4 focuses on unconscious processes in supervision.

The book goes on to explore the supervisor's tasks in relation to the learning and development of the supervisee (Chapter 5) and the importance of listening, exploration and interpretation (Chapter 6) in supervision. It goes on to consider the important and challenging issue of evaluation and assessment in supervision (Chapter 7) and the penultimate chapter (Chapter 8) focuses on ethics and supervision. The book ends with a consideration of supervision of supervision and a final reflection on being a supervisor.

The profession of supervision is complex and involves developing understanding and awareness in relation to a wide range of theories based on psychoanalytic, psychodynamic, systemic and supervisory principles and understandings. A vast range of literature is now available in the field and the references at the end of each chapter are a guide to many of them.

The chapters in this book cover the key issues that a supervisor needs to be aware of and consider. The supervisory examples are all based on supervisory experience but do not describe specific supervisees or their patients.

Acknowledgements

With grateful thanks to my professional colleague Stephen Crawford for his input and expertise on supervision and supervision training, my professional colleague Lynda Miller for reading the chapters and making insightful comments and suggestions and Stephen Driver for his editorial comments.

I would also like to thank all my colleagues and supervisees, especially those at WPF Therapy and the Society of Analytical Psychology, as they have all helped my ideas form and develop.

With thanks too, to Drs. Aner Govrin, Yael Peri Herzovich and Itamar Ezer for their invitation to write this book.

Chapter 1

Becoming and being a supervisor

Becoming a supervisor is a step into new and challenging areas of the profession and being a supervisor involves developing the capacity to process and manage complexity and requires additional and different skills to those of being a psychodynamic or psychoanalytic practitioner.[1] Becoming and being a supervisor entails acquiring a supervisory identity and supervisory mindedness (Watkins, 2018) and developing a supervisory analytic and reflective attitude in relation to the various layers of material presented in supervision, both conscious and unconscious, and making sense of them in relation to the patient material and the supervisee's development. It also requires developing supervisory agency and authority. This entails holding reflective integrity and responsibility in relation to the patient material, the work of the supervisee and the context and to discuss, explore, challenge, address issues and make decisions when necessary, in relation to the work and the requirements of the profession.

Historical background

The history of supervision reflects the growing recognition of the interplay of conscious and unconscious processes within supervision and the complexity of the supervisory relationship (Jacobs et al.,1995: Frawley-O'Dea, and Sarnat, 2001: Martin, 2002). In the early days of the psychoanalytic and psychotherapy profession, training copied 'the pattern of medical training' in that 'professional skills were acquired through work discussions with senior colleagues' (Martin, 2002:p.12) – a practice that Freud established at his Wednesday evening meetings,

DOI: 10.4324/9781003496137-1

which started in 1902. These meetings included discussion, but mainly involved Freud imparting information and theory in which the senior analyst, Freud, 'is in possession of knowledge and truth that is to be conveyed downward to the supervisee' (Frawley-O'Dea and Sarnat, 2001:p.16). Freud did advocate the need for 'self-examination' (Jacobs et al., 1995:p.12) in relation to clinical work but the Wednesday evening meetings primarily reflected a didactic format of supervision.

In 1913 Ferenczi set up the Budapest Psychoanalytic Society and established what became known as the Hungarian model of training in which the trainee's own analysis was the forum through which 'their thoughts, feelings and fantasies about their patients' (Martin, 2002:p.10) could be explored in a more dynamic and two-person way. In Berlin however, by the 1930s, the tripartite model of training, which we know today, became established and comprised training analysis, seminars and supervision, which included discussion but 'discouraged candidates from attending to their countertransference' (Frawley-O'Dea and Sarnat, 2001:p.21) and tended to retain a more didactic format.

It was not until the work of Paula Heimann (1949/50) on countertransference that a pathway opened up to consider unconscious dynamics and countertransference more fully within both therapy and supervision and led to Harold Searles (1955) and Ekstein and Wallerstein (1958) to develop a much fuller understanding of the conscious and unconscious dynamics of supervision. They identified that supervision is at least a three-person relationship of patient, therapist/supervisee and supervisor and recognised the importance of the supervisor's emotional experience, the dynamics of the reflection process (Searles, 1955), parallel process (see Chapter 4) and the impact of all aspects of the clinical rhombus on the supervisory dynamic (Figure 1.1) (Ekstein and Wallerstein, 1958), including the context.

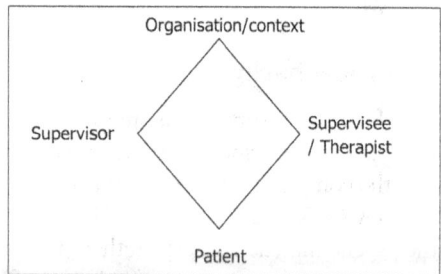

Figure 1.1 The Clinical Rhombus
Source: Ekstein, and Wallerstein, 1958:p.11.

Supervision therefore evolved from being primarily a one-person relationship of imparting information to one in which the supervisor needs to hold, reflect on, work with and within the triangular and four-fold dynamic of supervision. As a result, it became apparent that a supervisor needs to develop the capacity to consider, and reflect on, the impact of all of these processes within the supervisory relationship so as to create understanding in relation to the patient material and the learning needs of the supervisee.

However, for many years, supervision was primarily focused on training but as more counselling, psychotherapy and analytic trainings emerged in the 1960s, 70s and 80s onward the need for more supervisors arose and the need for training in supervision began to be identified. In the United Kingdom, trainings in supervision began in the 1980s but they were not widespread. Also, supervision after training as an analyst or psychotherapist was still not mandatory and so the need for supervision training remained limited. However, by the 1990s, in the United Kingdom, the push for supervision training began to be promoted by the professional bodies and by organisations such as WPF Therapy which offered supervision training and led to the setting up of the British Association of Psychoanalytic and Psychodynamic Supervision (BAPPS) in 1994. There was also increasing awareness of the complexity of supervision and books and papers on supervision (see references) began to grow. From the 1980s onwards there was also a growing recognition that supervision was needed post-qualification in order to develop the work with patients and unravel transference and countertransference issues and by the 2000s supervision post-qualification became a continuing professional development requirement in many countries, including the United Kingdom. Psychotherapy and counselling was also being offered in much wider contexts so the demand for supervision and trained supervisors increased. This resulted in many more supervision trainings being offered and the need for supervision training more widely acknowledged.

Supervision today

What is recognised today is that being a supervisor involves processing complexity. At one level it is a triangular dynamic between the patient, therapist/supervisee and supervisor or, as Gediman and Wolkenfeld (1980) describe a triadic intersubjective matrix. But supervision is also impacted on by all aspects of the clinical rhombus including the context. These all generate interactive processes which are conscious, unconscious, inter-personal and intra-psychic and need to be considered in relation to the work with the patient and the dynamics of the supervisory relationship (see Chapters 4 and 7) in order to 'understand the unfolding therapeutic reality' (Yerushalmi, 2024:p.26) of the work with the patient. This also involves the supervisor considering the learning needs of the supervisee (see Chapter 5) and be mindful of, and work with, issues of difference and diversity (see Chapter 3). The process of supervision can also facilitate change in the supervisee, which can help the patient change and gain insight (see Chapter 5).

Becoming a supervisor entails developing the capacity to contain and manage all aspects of the clinical rhombus and to hold, reflect on and work with the multi-layered input and unconscious manifestations of the patient's material, the supervisee's presentation and the experience of the supervisory relationship. In addition supervision involves developing the supervisee's work with the patient, enabling their professional development and upholding professional standards. A complex task.

The role of a supervisor

Providing a definition of supervision can help to identify the roles and tasks of a supervisor and supervision. Over the years supervision has been defined in a variety of ways. Bernard and Goodyear (1998) examine definitions and styles of supervision and comment that Ekstein and Wallerstein (1958)

> portrayed supervision as a teaching and learning process that gives particular emphasis to the relationships between and among patient, therapist, and supervisor and the processes

that interplay among them ... in order to develop under-standing ... and benefit future work with patients.

(p.17)

Mander (2002) states that supervision is 'a process of conceptualising and consulting with another mind' (p.39) and Zachrisson (2011) states that 'the aim of supervision is that a candidate (trainee) acquires psychoanalytic competence in a broad sense' (p.947). How-ever, supervision and being a supervisor requires a much wider and deeper definition in order to identify the roles, tasks and perspectives required of a supervisor in relation to the needs of the patient and the development of the supervisee.

The following definition of supervision evolved following research with a number of supervisors. They stated that super-vision needs to,

a   provide a boundaried and secure frame and a safe holding environment for in person or online supervision
b   hold the clinical rhombus (patient, therapist/supervisee, supervisor and context) and reflect on it in relation to the supervisory work
c   enable a space for reflection, thought and exploration in rela-tion to the patient material
d   reflect on unconscious communication and parallel process phenomena to enable the development of the clinical work and understanding of the patient
e   develop the work of the supervisee through supportive, infor-mative, explorative, analytic and reflective processes
f   enable the supervisee to evaluate the patient's needs, make hypotheses and develop a deeper understanding of the patient's inner world
g   enable the supervisee to deepen and develop their work with patients and transference, countertransference and uncon-scious processes
h   reflect on issues relating to race, culture, gender, difference and diversity etc., in relation to the clinical and supervisory work
i   enable the supervisee to identify when a patient requires a referral to other health professionals, e.g., a psychiatrist

j   evaluate the work of the supervisee and provide feedback in order to identify learning needs and/or fitness to practice issues

k   work with organisational requirements

l   uphold the professional and ethical requirements of the psychoanalytic and psychodynamic profession.

This list is extensive but not exhaustive because some issues, such as patient problems and supervisee learning needs, may overlap. A supervisor therefore needs to develop not only the capacity to identify the patient issues consciously presented in supervision but also reflect on what is unconsciously presented and what factors they relate to (see Chapters 4, 5 and 7). This requires a supervisor to be flexible and open in their attitude and approach and maintain an active reflective capacity in relation to the supervisee and the supervisee's presentations of patient material. It also requires a supervisor to hold an appropriate supervisory authority and be proactive when specific issues need to be addressed (see Chapter 8).

However, supervision is complex because the main focus of supervision, the patient, is absent (Martin, 2002) from the supervisory relationship and any information about the patient and the session(s) comes via the supervisee. As a result, the supervisor needs to consider the dynamics and transference and countertransference issues between the patient and therapist/supervisee and between the supervisee and themselves in relation to the patient material (see Chapter 4). In addition, a supervisor needs to consider any influences, conscious or unconscious, from the context of the clinical or supervisory work and the dynamics of the clinical rhombus to inform them of what might be impacting on the supervisory relationship and the clinical work. As Watkins (2014) comments, 'becoming a competent supervisor requires becoming grounded in the relational foundations that underlie the practice of psychoanalytic supervision' (p.225).

Being a supervisor

Being a supervisor therefore requires being able to multi-task internally and relationally in terms of the needs of the patient and the supervisee. This means that there are a number of areas and issues that need to be considered and identified by a supervisor, which this book covers, in order to offer effective supervision. They entail,

a   setting the contract and boundaries for the supervision work in relation to the supervisee's clinical work and any organisational/context issues
b   creating a supervisory alliance
c   working with the supervisee to consider the patient's issues and the therapeutic encounter
d   considering unconscious processes in supervision so as to develop awareness and understanding of any parallel processes and unconscious communication in relation to the patient and the learning needs of the supervisee
e   utilising exploratory dialogue and interpretive skills so as to engage the supervisee in developing understanding about the patient and the patient's internal world
f   identifying the learning needs of the supervisee and developing the supervisee's capacity to work psychodynamically or psychoanalytically
g   evaluating and assessing the capabilities of a supervisee in relation to training or professional requirements
h   being proactive when required in relation to supervisory issues
i   working with issues of race, culture, gender and intersectionality in relation to the patient material and supervisor processes
j   upholding ethical principles and the standards of the profession and addressing them if areas of concerns or fitness to practice issues arise with a supervisee
k   finding authority and humility (Watkins and Hook, 2016) from which to work and relate to the needs of the patient and the learning needs of the supervisee.

Roth and Pilling (2015) provide a detailed account of the skills and competencies required to be a supervisor, which range from generic ones to specific and meta competencies in relation to patient issues, supervisee learning needs and ethics. But being a supervisor is not just a tick box of tasks. It requires a relational capacity to contain, hold and actively engage the supervisee in exploration and understanding about the patient. This is important because the patient is only heard and experienced through the presentation of the supervisee. A supervisor therefore needs to develop 'mutual exploration, mutual wonder, a dialogue in which neither participant always knows which is the best tack to take, but in which the two make discoveries together that ultimately help both the patient and therapist find their own voices' (Jacobs, David and Meyer, 1995:p.29).

Finding a meta-perspective

The supervisory container is complex because it contains the interplay of many factors. The main focus may be the patient but issues from all aspects of the clinical rhombus intermingle and interact in the inter-active field of supervision. Being a supervisor therefore requires developing the capacity to consider the multi-layered, conscious and unconscious, interactive processes and communications inherent in supervision. In order to achieve, from time to time, a meta-perspective (Figure 1.2) in relation to the issues impacting on the supervisory work a supervisor needs to develop their observing ego (Greenson, 1981) and maintain an analytic and self-reflecting attitude, which rotates through, and reflects on, all aspects of the clinical rhombus (see Chapters 4, 5 and 7) in order to generate understanding about the patient and the work

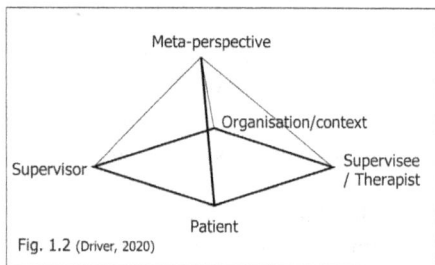

Fig. 1.2 (Driver, 2020)

Figure 1.2 A Meta-perspective
Source: Author (2020).

of the supervisee (Driver, 2020:p.131). Such reflective and exploratory processes also enable the supervisee to develop and deepen their understanding of the dynamics of the work with the patient and the patient's internal world.

Final comment

Therapists who become supervisors are both beginners and have experience. The challenge is to translate the skill set of being a therapist into becoming a supervisor and taking on board the additional skills and understandings that being a supervisor requires. Becoming a supervisor involves considering and exploring the theories of supervision in relation to the conscious, unconscious and interactional processes inherent in supervision. It also includes learning how to process the complex interactional field of supervision such as parallel process (see Chapter 4) and transference and countertransference in relation to the patient material, the supervisee or both. Learning how to unravel, process and reflect on these dynamics so as to enable a greater understanding of the patient, the development of the work of a supervisee and uphold professional standards is fundamental to being a supervisor. The chapters in this book take you through the skills, theories and issues that becoming and being a supervisor entails.

Note

1 In this book I use both psychoanalytic and psychodynamic titles because both terms reflect the spectrum of practitioners who work with transference, countertransference and the dynamics of the unconscious.

References

Bernard, J.M. and Goodyear, R.K. (1998) *Fundamentals of Clinical Supervision. Second Edition*. London and Toronto: Allyn and Bacon.

Driver, C. (2020) *The Self and the Quintessence*. London and New York: Routledge.

Ekstein, R., and Wallerstein, R.S. (1958) *The Teaching and Learning of Psychotherapy*. Madison Connecticut: International Universities Press, Inc.

Frawley-O'Dea, M.G. and Sarnat, J.E. (2001) *The Supervisory Relationship*. New York: The Guilford Press.

Gediman H., and Wolkenfeld, F. (1980) 'The parallelism phenomenon in psychoanalysis and supervision: Its reconsideration as a triadic system'. *Psychoanal. Q.* (49):234–255.

Greenson, R.R. (1981) *The Technique and Practice of Psychoanalysis*. London: Hogarth Press.

Heimann, P. (1949/50) 'On countertransference'. Tonnesmann, M. (ed) (1989) *About Children and Children No-Longer. Collected Papers.* London: Routledge.

Jacobs, D., David, P., and Meyer, D.J. (1995) *The Supervisory Encounter.* New Haven and London: Yale University.

Mander, G. (2002) 'Supervision: Between control and collusion'. Driver, C., and Martin, E. (eds.) *Supervising Psychotherapy.* London: Sage Publications.

Martin, E. (2002) 'Listening to the absent patient'. Driver, C., and Martin, E. (eds.) *Supervising Psychotherapy.* London: Sage Publications.

Roth, A.D., and Pilling, S. (2015) 'A competence framework for the supervision of psychological therapies'. Research Department of Clinical, Educational and Health Psychology. University College London. https://www.ucl.ac.uk/pals/sites/pals/files/background_document_sup ervision_competences_july_2015.pdf (Accessed 23. 03. 2024).

Searles, H.F. (1955) 'The informational value of the supervisor's emotional experiences'. Searles, H.F. (1986) *Collected Papers on Schizophrenia and Related Subjects.* London: Maresfield Library.

Watkins, C.E. (2014) 'The competent psychoanalytic supervisor: Some thoughts about supervision competences for accountable practice and training'. *Int. Forum Psychoanal.* (23)(4):220–228.

Watkins, C.E. (2018) 'Being and becoming a psychotherapy supervisor: The crucial triad of learning difficulties'. *Am. J. of Psychother.* 30 Apr 2018. https://doi.org/10.1176/appi.psychotherapy.2013.67.2.135.

Watkins, C.E., and Hook, J. (2016) 'On a Culturally Humble Psychoanalytic Supervision Perspective: Creating the Cultural Third'. *Psychoanal. Psychol.* (33)(3):487–517.

Yerushalmi, H. (2024) 'Future developments in psychoanalytic supervision'. *Psychodynamic Practice* (30)(1):19–29.

Zachrisson, A. (2011) 'Dynamics of psychoanalytic supervision: A heuristic model'. *Int. J. Psychoanal.* (92)(4):943–961.

Chapter 2

The supervisory container

Understanding and identifying the factors needed to create and develop a safe supervisory container for the exploration of the clinical work and the development of the supervisee is a vital initial step in the process of supervision. This requires consideration of the contract with the supervisee, frames and boundaries, the roles and tasks of being a supervisor and understanding the dynamics inherent within supervision. This includes holding and reflecting on the conscious and unconscious impact of internal processes and external factors on the supervisory frame and the supervisory processes.

The contract

The first step in setting up a supervisory relationship, group or individual, is to identify and agree a contract with the supervisee(s) and be aware that there are both conscious and unconscious reasons why the contract and frame are important. A safe and boundaried supervisory contract requires a supervisor to define:

- the context: in person or online
- time
- frequency
- boundaries
- fee, and whether missed supervisory sessions are paid for
- confidentiality.

DOI: 10.4324/9781003496137-2

In group supervision it is also helpful to create an understanding and contract between the group members about how they will work together and agree confidentiality in relation to what it presented in the group (see also Chapter 3). Within an agency setting there may be other aspects of the contract which will need to be clarified and agreed such as completing organisational administration, etc.

In addition it is important to discuss the following when setting up the contract:

- the type of work to be supervised
- confidentiality in relation to in person or online work
- clinical responsibility and accountability
- type of supervision to be offered, e.g., training supervision, supervision for qualified practitioners, peer supervision, managerial or consultancy supervision
- difference and diversity
- training requirements and whether reports are required
- evaluation
- procedures for emergencies and contact outside of the supervisory hour if an emergency arises.

Different contractual arrangements will also need to be defined in relation to each context (in person, online, private practice or organisational). This is especially important around issues of confidentiality. When supervising, confidentiality relates to what is spoken about but it is important to clarify when confidentiality might need to be broken such as if a safeguarding issue is identified. For online supervision issues about confidentiality are more complex because it often takes place outside of a consulting room. It is therefore important for the supervisor to model a contained and boundaried online space and confirm and agree with the supervisee that any online work occurs within a confidential space that will not be interrupted by family or other people and that what is spoken about is confidential.

Setting the contract sets the frame and clarifies the parameters of the work. As well as discussing and agreeing these issues openly it is also helpful to have a short, written, contract with a supervisee so that what is agreed is recorded and understood by both supervisor and supervisee(s). In addition, it is also important to confirm that a supervisee has a contract with their patients and that the therapy occurs in a contained and confidential space, in person or online, and if online that their patients call in from a space which is contained and confidential for them.

A supervisor needs to be proactive in establishing the contract and ground rules of the supervision so that both supervisor and supervisee(s) understand the frame and parameters of how they will work together. The contract creates a clearly defined space from which to consider, explore and understand the patient material presented and enable the development of the supervisee.

Frames and boundaries

Supervision is the container into which the work with the patient is considered and the development of the supervisee enabled. It is therefore important to consider the frame in relation to this. The boundaries of the supervisory frame are created by the time, place and setting but they are also created and influenced by how the supervisor relates within the frame (see Chapter 3). Yerushalmi (2018) comments that 'when the supervisory setting is stable, clear, and safe, it enables the supervisee and supervisor to reflect upon their subjective contributions, as well as on the intersubjective processes in therapy' (p.233). In addition Ogden (2005) argues that 'the supervisor is responsible for creating a frame that ensures the supervisee's freedom to think and dream and be alive to what is occurring both in the analytic process and in the supervisory process' (p.1269). However, it is important for a supervisor to be aware that the unconscious is always present within the supervisory relationship and that we do not always operate from 'ego-oriented states' (Gee, 2003:p.164). Wood (2007) reflects that 'we are all subject to unconscious forces that may compromise our professionalism' (p.25) and that, when necessary, these need to be considered in relation to boundaries in supervision. (See also Chapters 5 and 8).

It is also important to recognise the interconnection between the supervisory frame and the therapeutic relationship of therapist and patient. Langs (1994) identifies that the therapeutic relationship and the supervisory one are linked in a systemic way and that changes in one relationship has an impact on the other, consciously and unconsciously. For Langs (1994) changes to the supervisory frame impact on both supervisee and patient and result in overt or symbolic (encoded) communications which are important to understand and decode in supervision in relation to the patient material. As a result Langs considers that it is important to consider the impact of any frame changes on the patient material and the supervisory process because, he maintains, 'the frame exerts a strong influence over the conscious and unconscious experience and the functioning of the members of the system' (p.59).

Although strict adherence to the supervisory frame in the way Langs proposes may not always be possible what he is advocating, and which supervisors need to be mindful of, is that frame changes in supervision will have an impact on the work of the supervisee. For example constant changes to the time of supervision by the supervisor may convey to the supervisee a lack of respect for the frame and possibly lead to the supervisee/therapist changing the time of sessions with their patients. Offering cups of tea in supervision and personal conversations within supervision can convey a lack of appreciation for unconscious communication and diminish the focus on the patient material being brought into supervision. The questions that are helpful to ask when changes to the frame occur, which sometimes are inevitable, are "why do I need to change the frame?" and "what is the impact of the frame changes on the supervisee and the patient?"

A secure frame enables the supervisee to feel held, contained and provides a safe space for the clinical issues to be explored. But, Jacobs et al. (1995) outlines how, if boundaries are held too tightly, this can act as a defence against self-reflection (p.44) especially when issues arise in relation to the frame. When this occurs it requires careful and sensitive exploration by the supervisor. For example, when there has been a change of supervisor within an organisation a new supervisor might be viewed with suspicion, or a supervisee might be caught up in feelings of loss in relation to the previous supervisor. It is helpful, therefore, for the supervisor to be aware of, and perhaps discuss, such issues so as to clarify what is being brought into the supervisory frame by the supervisee(s).

Frequency and time in supervision

The frequency of supervision, what is brought to supervision and how it is presented is also important to consider and may depend on how many patients a supervisee is working with. A supervisee who holds a full caseload may need weekly supervision whereas someone only seeing two or three patients a week, and who is an experienced clinician, may only need to come monthly. In group supervision the frequency may depend on how many patients the group holds. However, often group supervision occurs in an organisational setting and the frequency is set by the organisation so the overall group caseload may need to be thought about and discussed.

The division of time in supervision also requires consideration. If a supervisee presents all their cases in a fifty-minute supervision session this gives an overview of their work but little time for in-depth exploration. Using the supervision time to explore one patient in detail provides the supervisee with a deeper, and potentially more insightful, process. In group supervision thought needs to be given to the time allocated for the presentation of each patient and also for each supervisee and it is containing for supervisees in a group to be given a clear time to present. In a one-and-a-half-hour supervision group of four supervisees I would normally allocate two supervisees to present one patient each supervision session. This does mean that the supervisees only present on alternate sessions, but allows time for more detailed exploration and, in a group, the supervisees also learn from each other. Of course, from time to time, emergencies arise, or clarification is sought, by a supervisee in relation to a patient and/or organisational issues and time needs to be given to explore and consider them. But overall it is holding and containing if there is a clear allocation of time in relation to both group and individual supervision.

Notes

A further question to consider relates to how the supervisee presents their work in supervision and what is helpful for you, as a supervisor, to know and hear about to enable exploration about the patient and develop the work of the supervisee.

Verbatim session notes of all or part of a session are often required by training organisations. These provide a detailed insight into what the patient talked about, how the supervisee responded, insight into how the supervisee works, the process of the session and how the patient responded after an intervention by the therapist/supervisee. In some settings the use of audio or video recordings are advocated or required. These require agreement by the patient but do provide detailed information about the content and interactions in the session and can be useful to track themes and the supervisee's way of working. Kernberg (2010) comments that

> detailed written material, drawn from written notes or audio recordings … provides a more accurate reflection of the dialogue and of the therapist's interventions, but may miss some of the subtleties of emotional interactions that are communicated by means of the parallel process.

(p.621)

Crawford (2005) considers that although verbatim notes

> can never fully capture the session as it was, they can give some idea of how the supervisee experiences and processes a session, and can provide a basis for free association, both in the writing of it and in the presenting of it in supervision.

(p.62)

However, verbatim notes and audio or video recordings can remain very two-dimensional and avoid consideration of the deeper unconscious communications inherent in the therapy sessions. Crawford (2005) advocates the use of process reports because they 'give a sense of the flow of the session, who said what, when and what was the response?' (p.62). This provides flexibility to allow discussion and free association in relation to the patient material and the work with the patient.

Flexibility about how the patient material and sessions are presented can enable more free flowing exploration and associations to transference and countertransference phenomena and unconscious communications. This can enable and deepen the supervisee's cognitive, perceptual and emotional understanding about the patient's internal world. Bernard and Goodyear (1998), citing research, comment that what is presented and how it is presented 'should be based on the immediate learning needs of the supervisee and that supervisors need to avoid fixed styles in their supervision' (p.93). In addition, what a supervisee presents always contains both manifest and latent content in relation to the patient, the session and the supervisor. This is because supervision is always formed of the 'psyches of patient, supervisee and supervisor' (Martin, 2002:p.15). What a supervisor needs to consider, therefore, is what style of presentation and exploration is helpful for the supervisee so that they can unravel the patient material and gain insight and understanding about the patient.

As a supervisor you may want to consider taking notes during the supervision session to keep track of the patient material, the supervisee's work, the process of the session(s) presented and your own thoughts and associations. This can be helpful so as to hold the many layers of material presented, provided it doesn't get in the way of the interaction and exploration with the supervisee.

Whatever notes are taken and kept it is important to know their legal status in relation to patient access. Written notes taken by supervisees or supervisors for their personal use cannot normally be requested to be seen by the patient but should be destroyed when not needed. Any notes or records kept on computer databases should be factual only and not relate to hypotheses about transference and countertransference, etc. Session records, within the United Kingdom, can be requested and accessed by the patient. It is important for a supervisor, or an organisation, to know the legal status and data-protection regulations regarding notes and records.

The supervisory container

For a supervisor to understand and evaluate what they are dealing with (see also Chapter 7) it is helpful to identify the elements and issues that are being brought into supervision. This requires a proactive stance by the supervisor to gain the information needed to inform them of the work that they are supervising. The information that is helpful for a supervisor to know about in relation to the supervisee is:

- Where did the supervisee train?
- The level of training and experience of the supervisee?
- How much experience of clinical work does the supervisee have?
- How much personal therapy has the supervisee had?
- Is the supervisee currently in therapy?
- What professional organisation does the supervisee belong to?
- Where does the supervisee work – privately and/or in an organisation?
- What is the organisation that they work for and what type of clinical work does it offer?
- How many patients is the supervisee seeing each week and what is the frequency of patients?

In relation to the patients being presented it is helpful to have background information so as to orientate perception and understanding. Mander (2002) comments,

> what I really prefer is a profile of each patient which I use as a *aide-mémoire* during the presentation and which miraculously turns into an Ariadne's thread, guiding me into, around and out of the maze of each individual's life story, a template into which I fit the detail of the presentation.
>
> (p.147)

It is therefore important to identify the information needed to enable the generation of understanding about the patient. In relation to the patient(s) presented it is helpful to know:

- the age, gender and family background of the patient
- the patient's personal and relationship history
- the patient's current life situation
- the presenting problem that has brought the patient to therapy.

Obtaining such information about the supervisee, the patient and the context enables the supervisor to gather up the issues that they are holding, containing and working with.

The supervisory container includes the conscious and unconscious dynamics emanating from the patient, the supervisee/therapist, the supervisor and the context or organisation in which the clinical work is taking place; a dynamic that Ekstein and Wallerstein (1958) called the clinical rhombus (see Chapters 1 and 3). Supervision is a relational activity, which aims to understand and develop the work with the patient and enable the development of the supervisee, but it is also a system in which input and changes in one aspect affects other aspects of it. The supervisory container, which the supervisor is providing, is therefore physical, internal, inter-personal and intra-psychic.

The dynamics of the container

The main aim in creating a contained and boundaried space within supervision is so that exploration of the patient's issues and the work of the supervisee can evolve. However, sometimes the presentation of the patient material recreates the dynamics and issues that the patient has brought to the therapist/supervisee and creates a parallel process in supervision (see Chapter 4). Mattinson (1975) speaks of the supervisory relationship as being a seamless web with the therapeutic one because the therapeutic relationship is contained within the supervisory one. Hawkins and Shohet (2002) describe a 'double matrix' (p.69) model of supervision. Here the clinical rhombus of supervisor, supervisee/therapist, patient and context is considered in terms of the overlapping matrices of the therapeutic system and the supervisory system. Their model identifies how supervision can focus attention on any aspect of the matrix such as the patient, the therapist/supervisee, transference and countertransference, the fantasy relationship, conscious and unconscious dynamics and the context in which the supervision occurs. Such processes requires a supervisor to develop a 'helicopter ability' (Hawkins and Shohet, 2002:p. 44) from which they can hover, dip in and out of exploring the different dynamics and interactions and develop understanding with the supervisee. Perry (2003) introduces the concept of the supervisory matrix which 'offers a framework for thinking about the multiplicity of relationships and meanings in supervision' (p.202). Within this supervisory matrix there is a constant interaction and emergence of affects, countertransference, transference from all participants which, in supervision, generates the potential for free association, synthesis, understanding, 'meaning and mutual growth for both patient and therapist' (p.203).

These models identify how supervision is a multi-layered and complex web of conscious and unconscious communication communicated through projection, projective identification, transference, countertransference and the dynamics inherent in a relationship. This means that the supervisory relationship becomes the container for the unconscious communication of raw and unprocessed thoughts, feelings and affects emanating from the therapeutic relationship and the patient material. It is the role of the supervisor to hold and contain these dynamics so that they can be processed, thought about and understood.

The supervisory context

Another factor to consider is the context of the supervision. Supervision within an organisation or a context focusing on specific patient issues such as eating disorders, torture, abuse, rape, etc., may involve specific areas of expertise and understanding which may require a supervisor to learn more about a particular field of clinical work. Supervising trainees (see Chapter 5) may require utilising different supervisory styles to enable learning whereas exploration of unconscious processes and transference and countertransference will be easier when supervising more experienced and qualified supervisees. Supervision in private practice brings with it issues of responsibility in relation to the supervisory work. The question to consider is, what types of supervision do you do and what is the impact of the context on the work?

Within an organisational context the supervisory container can also have multifaceted dimensions, which a supervisor needs to be aware of and consider. As Hawkins and Shohet (2002) comment 'all helping organizations are, by their very nature, importing

distress, disturbance, fragmentation and need' in which the clinicians 'if they are empathically relating to the client's distress, will
experience parallel distress and sometimes disturbance and fragmentation within themselves' (p.153). For a supervisor it is
important, therefore, to not only consider the impact of the organization and the patient group on the supervisee but also the
impact on themselves (see Chapter 3). In addition, it is sometimes
the case that an organisation becomes dysfunctional due to staff
changes, lack of leadership or the organisational culture. In such
situations the supervisor may feel torn between their supervision
of their supervisees and "supervising" the organisation and/or
becoming directly involved in the organisational management.
Whilst this is sometimes inevitable it is important that a supervisor remains aware of what they are being pulled into and consider their own limitations so that they can maintain a focused
and safe supervisory space in which to consider the clinical material and the needs of the supervisee.

Holding

Containment and holding may seem very similar concepts but, as
Ogden (2004) points out, the concept of holding, derived from
Winnicott's work, has a more ontological meaning and relates to
the 'qualities of the experience' (p.1350). Holding is about security,
continuity, consistency and trust experienced over time and 'fosters
self- and object constancy' (McWilliams, 2021:p.52) in relation to
the supervisory alliance and the clinical work presented. The
experience of supervision for both supervisor and supervisee may,
and inevitably will, change depending on the patient being presented or circumstances – both internal and external – but holding
a space for consideration of the clinical work and the supervisee's
experience generates a safe space for thought and reflection.

An example of this was the impact of the Covid pandemic,
lockdowns and the sudden end of in person meetings, which had
been the mainstay of therapeutic and supervisory work. The rapid
adaption by the profession to the use of online meetings via
Zoom, Teams, Skype, Phone, etc., provided an ongoing continuity
of the secure, holding and reflective space that a supervisor and

supervision provides. As McWilliams (2021) identifies a 'secure relational base' (p.58) is integral to the holding environment of supervision and creates a space for reflection, the development of a reflective ego and the internalisation of the supervisory perspective. A process which mirrors and reflects to the supervisee how they can be with their patients.

However, the holding environment of supervision is not just about providing security and consistency, it is also about developing trust. Trust in supervision develops from the supervisory relationship and the supervisory alliance as well as the competencies and attitude of the supervisor. Watkins (2013) comments on the importance of a supervisory relationship 'characterized by supervisor empathy and respect and built on trust and confidentiality' (p.625). This is important because supervision is exposing for the supervisee and they often need to share difficult and possibly shame-inducing experiences that have emerged in the work with their patients. Trust that the supervisor will provide a safe and ego-based reflective space and not a frightening persecutory superego one will enable the supervisee to bring and explore the difficulties and uncertainties that clinical work often generates. Sometimes, however, a supervisee will need to be challenged when things have gone wrong, or their work is not fit for practice or unethical. But trust in a safe exploratory space is vital in creating a holding environment which can enable the supervisee to explore, reflect and think.

The supervisory frame and the external world

What has been described above is an ideal scenario of a contained frame in which thinking and processing can occur. However, the realities of clinical work mean that sometimes the supervisory frame needs to be opened out to others. Sometimes in clinical work safeguarding issues emerge which require contacting external agencies such as social services or the police. When there is a suicide risk or other medical concerns the patient's doctor may need to be contacted. All of these issues require careful consideration in relation to the process, confidentiality and patient consent. This may require the supervisor to seek supervision or advice for themselves.

If the supervisee is a trainee a supervisor often needs to write reports for the training organisation. If there are ethical or fitness to practice concerns about the work of the supervisee then the supervisor might need to contact the ethics committee of the organisation in which the supervisee is registered. In such scenarios the supervisor needs to consider a number of issues: 'the organisational or training requirements, the learning experience of the supervisee' (Stewart, 2002:p.78), the needs of the patient and the requirements of the law and/or the profession.

Such situations create anxiety for both supervisor and supervisee and may require the supervisor to seek advice or supervision of supervision so that they can process what is presented and how they need to respond. Supervision cannot always be a sealed container as it needs to hold and acknowledge both internal and external realities. However, the key role that a supervisor provides is a place to process, reflect and think so that when the frame is opened up it is done so with thought and understanding.

Final reflection

The creation of a safe space by the supervisor and the holding and containing function of supervision and the supervisory relationship is an important step in creating a working alliance and a creative space to process and think about the patient material with the supervisee. As Ungar and Ahumada (2001) argue, the key function of supervision 'is to help contain the emotional turbulence and unconscious anxieties arising and evolving in the analytic and supervisory sessions' so that 'the therapist-patient interaction and that of the supervisee and supervisor can be understood as twin, tiered transformational arenas' (p.71). Within this the role of the supervisor and the process of supervision is at the service of the clinical work with the patient and the development of the supervisee. For this to occur the supervisor needs to provide a safe container in which the patient material and the dynamics with the therapist/supervisee can emerge.

References

Bernard, J.M. and Goodyear, R.K. (1998) *Fundamentals of Clinical Supervision. Second Edition.* London and Toronto: Allyn and Bacon.

Crawford, S. (2005) 'Free association and supervision'. Driver, C., and Martin, E. (eds.) *Supervision and the Analytic Attitude.* London: Whurr.

Ekstein, R. and Wallerstein, R.S. (1958) *The Teaching and Learning of Psychotherapy.* Madison Connecticut: International Universities Press, Inc.

Gee, H. (2003) 'Boundaries in supervision'. Wiener, J., Mizen, R. and Duckham, J. (eds.) *Supervision and Being Supervised: A Practice in Search of a Theory.* Basingstoke: Palgrave Macmillan.

Hawkins, P. and Shohet, R. (2002) *Supervision in the Helping Professions,* 2nd edition. Buckingham and Philadelphia: Open University Press.

Jacobs, D., David, P., and Meyer, D.J. (1995) *The Supervisory Encounter.* New Haven and London: Yale University.

Kernberg, O. F. (2010) 'Psychoanalytic supervision: The supervisor's tasks'. *Psychoanal. Q.,* (79)(3):603–627.

Langs, R. (1994) *Doing Supervision and Being Supervised.* London: Karnac Books.

Mander, G. (2002) 'Timing and ending in supervision'. Driver, C., and Martin, E. (eds.) *Supervising Psychotherapy.* London: Sage Publications.

Martin, E. (2002) 'Listening to the absent patient'. Driver, C., and Martin, E. (eds.) *Supervising Psychotherapy.* London: Sage Publications.

Mattinson, J. (1975) *The Reflection Process in Casework Supervision.* London: Tavistock Institute of Marital Studies.

McWilliams, N. (2021) *Psychoanalytic Supervision.* New York and London: The Guilford Press.

Ogden, T.H. (2004) 'On holding and containing, being and dreaming'. *Int. J. of Psychoanal.* 85:1349–1364.

Ogden, T. (2005) 'On psychoanalytic supervision'. *Int. J. Psychoanal.* (86)(5):1265–1280.

Perry, C. (2003) 'Into the labyrinth: A developing approach to supervision'. Wiener, J., Mizen, R. and Duckham, J. (eds.) *Supervision and Being Supervised: A Practice in Search of a Theory.* Basingstoke: Palgrave Macmillan.

Stewart, J. (2002) 'The container and the contained: Supervision and its organisational context'. Driver, C. and Martin, E. (eds.) *Supervising Psychotherapy.* London: Sage Publications.

Ungar, V. and Ahumada, L. (2001) 'Supervision. A container-contained approach'. *Int. J. Psychoanal.* (82)(1):71–81.

Watkins, C.E. (2013) 'On psychoanalytic supervisor competencies, the persistent paradox without parallel in psychoanalytic education, and dreaming of an evidence-based psychoanalytic supervision'. *Psychoanal. Rev.* (100)(4):609–646.

Wood, H. (2007) 'Boundaries and confidentiality in supervision'. Petts, A. and Shapley, B. (eds) *On Supervision. Psychoanalytic and Jungian Analytic Perspectives.* London: Karnac.

Yerushalmi, H. (2018) 'Loneliness, Closeness and Shared Responsibility in Supervision'. *Am. J. Psychoanal.* (78)(3):231–246.

Chapter 3

The supervisory relationship

Supervision is a relational activity in which the therapeutic relationship (patient and therapist/supervisee) sits within the supervisory one. Supervision is also a process which is influenced by the attitude of the supervisor and how they work with the supervisee to understand the patient and develop the supervisee's clinical skills and internal capacity to process conscious and unconscious communication. The processes of supervision require an interactive dialogue between supervisor and supervisee and this depends on the supervisory alliance.

The supervisory alliance

Supervision is exposing. It exposes the patient but it also exposes the supervisee and their work. Crawford (2005) comments, 'supervisees have to be able to tolerate letting supervisors know about their working relationships with patients and what goes on in their consulting rooms' (p.59). In addition anxieties and projections can creep into the supervisory relationship and affect what is brought and why it is brought. It is therefore important, as a supervisor, to be aware that the processes of supervision rely heavily on the development of a supervisory alliance. Watkins (2014) concludes that the supervisory alliance is vital in relation to the work with the patient and the development of the supervisee and he points out that a good supervisory alliance leads to,

DOI: 10.4324/9781003496137-3

higher supervisee self-efficacy and well-being, greater willingness to self-disclose during supervision, more satisfaction with supervision, ... and greater perceived effectiveness of supervision.

(p.41)

In contrast a poor supervisory alliance was found to be related to,

Supervisee avoidant attachment style, higher degree of perceived stress, more exhaustion and burnout, greater amount of role conflict and role ambiguity, and more frequently perceived occurrences of negative supervision events.

(p.41)

The development of the supervisory alliance is therefore vital for effective supervision because supervision requires openness, rapport, a willingness to collaborate and explore, an openness to learning and the capacity to use the self, by both supervisee and supervisor, in relation to the exploration of the patient material. Creating this alliance is part of the challenge of being a supervisor because supervisees (and supervisors) come to any relationship with pre-conceptions, superego perspectives and transference issues. Being aware of the factors that can influence, generate or hinder a good working relationship is part of the supervisor's role so as to ensure that the needs of the patient and the learning needs of the supervisee are maintained.

Establishing the supervisory alliance

Establishing the supervisory alliance is rarely an immediate process and depends on the context of the supervision and the internal world of both supervisee and supervisor. In a training setting supervisees and supervisors often do not choose who they see so both are stepping into an unknown. This may result in supervisees in training having preconceptions about the supervisor based on their own internal issues, fears and anxieties about being judged and found wanting and the myths and stories that surround a particular supervisor, all of which will affect their attitude to the supervisor and supervision. In addition, a supervisor may have their preconceptions about a supervisee based on reports or feedback from the training.

In an organisational setting preconceptions and anxieties may be present but, in addition, the supervisee and supervisor will need to fit into the requirements and culture of the organisation and the patient groups. Qualified practitioners working in private practice are normally able to choose a supervisor but the choice may not be straightforward and transference issues may be involved. In addition, what a supervisee wants from supervision may not always match what a supervisor assumes they want (Nagell et al., 2014). A supervisor therefore needs to be aware that underlying intra-psychic, inter-personal and organisational dynamics will affect the development of the supervisory alliance. So, the start of a supervisory relationship may begin in an hesitant and defensive way due to anxiety, vulnerability, preconceptions and uncertainty within both supervisee and supervisor. What needs to evolve is a secure base and a secure relationship between supervisee and supervisor so that an open exploratory space can be formed, and the supervisory alliance developed.

It is clear that a secure and contained supervisory space is important for the development of the supervisory alliance so that the supervisee can 'feel supported in their explorations' (Driver, 2005:p.71). The supervisory alliance also develops as trust, collaboration and supervisee development progresses. At the start of a supervisory relationship the supervisory alliance may be fragile and require the supervisor to take the lead in creating an exploratory alliance in relation to the patient material. Nagell et al., (2014) comment that the 'supervision relationship develops with time' (p.575) but that 'at the beginning of the supervisory work there should be a joint understanding and agreement about what the form and content should be, as well as the specific working method of the supervisor' (p.576). Time therefore needs to be given to identify how the supervisor and supervisee will work together and develop a supervisory alliance in which both supervisee and supervisor are mutually engaged in processes of exploration, reflection and understanding. Brown and Miller (2002) comment that 'when the supervisory alliance has sufficiently matured and the candidate's self-esteem as an analyst is more solidified so that he/she has a mind of his/her own, then he/she is better able to engage in a less defensive examination of experiences in the supervisory relationship' (p.814) and make use of the self in this process.

Watkins (2012) considers that the real relationship between supervisee and supervisor is also important (p.252) because unless the supervisee feels free to talk about significant life issues in supervision the supervisory process may be impeded or stagnate. For example, a supervisee who has had a recent bereavement may find it hard to explore issues relating to loss and bereavement with a patient or with the supervisor. If the supervisor is aware of the supervisee's loss this can be sensitively and empathically acknowledged and held until the supervisee is ready to explore the patient issues in more depth. The real relationship is important, but it also needs to be in the service of the clinical work in terms of what might be affecting the supervisee at a particular point in time. Overall, the alliance and the relationship between the supervisor and supervisee needs to be subsumed to a focus on the patient along with the professional development of the supervisee (see Chapter 5).

The development of the alliance also depends on the style and manner of interaction and communication by the supervisor (see Chapter 6), the level of development and experience of the supervisee (see Chapter 5 and 7) and the degree to which anxiety and superego dynamics affect the supervisory relationship. A didactic and critical supervisor will create an anxiety-based supervisory relationship that is not conducive to the development of a supervisory alliance. A secure base, trust and an open, exploratory and collaborative style of supervision, in which there is an empathic appreciation of the challenges of analytic and psychodynamic work, will generate in the supervisee a feeling of being held and understood in a safe container. This will enable a supervisee to gradually form a supervisory alliance with the supervisor, facilitate mutual exploration and enable the 'supervisee to develop their own identity as therapists' (Driver, 2002a:p.57).

Establishing a supervisory alliance is important because without it the inter-personal and intra-psychic explorations that are fundamental to the processes of psychoanalytic or psychodynamic supervision are impeded and understanding about the patient and the development of the supervisee limited. However a supervisor also needs to be mindful of the danger of the supervisory relationship becoming either one of 'control or collusion' (Mander, 2002a:p.39). For Mander when a supervisor becomes controlling they are ignoring the presence of the supervisee and when colluding the presence of the patient. Either approach disregards the triangular dynamic of supervision and impedes independent thinking and exploration by the supervisee. Occasionally, however, a supervisor does need to use their authority but needs to be mindful of their power and not use it inappropriately to control the supervisee.

Overall, the aim of a good supervisory alliance is the development of a collaborative relationship in which curiosity and creative exploration, both inter-personal and intra-psychic, can take place about the patient and the dynamics of the therapeutic work. In addition, it facilitates the capacity to hold and reflect on the multiple variables that clinical and supervisory work entail. A vital internal skill for both therapist and supervisor. When a supervisee feels held, contained and heard, the supervisory alliance enables ego-to-ego relating between supervisee and supervisor, an openness to learning and the development of the supervisee's internal reflective function and reverie about the patient.

The supervisory alliance and the context of supervision

The context in which the clinical work and/or supervision takes place will also affect the supervisory alliance. In private practice both therapist and supervisor have more control over the frame and contract of the therapeutic or supervisory work in terms of patients or supervisees seen, time, fees, context and contracts. In an organisational context there are organisational parameters to consider which will impact on both the therapeutic and supervisory work.

Organisations create a culture and system that staff are required to adhere to and normally will set the contract, fee and the length of time patients are seen. In addition, an organisation will develop policies and procedures and implement changes to adapt to internal or external requirements (Stewart, 2002b:p.108). When organisational changes occur they ripple through the clinical rhombus and affect the patient, therapist/supervisee and supervisor. When, for example, an organisation changes its fees this impacts on, and stirs up, transference and countertransference dynamics in all parties. In such a situation a supervisor will need to process their own feelings and enable the supervisee to self-process (Langs, 1994) theirs in order to unearth and understand the particular ways that such changes have affected the patient and what they present.

The specific culture, focus or patient group will also have an impact on supervision. Organisations offering counselling or therapy to victims of domestic abuse, refugees, torture, etc., see patients who bring to the therapy, overtly or covertly, the violence of their experience. This has an impact on the therapist which is then brought into supervision. Supervisors need to be aware of their countertransference and the effect of such work because of the real danger of vicarious traumatisation. This requires sensitivity and awareness to ensure that the work is not negatively impacting on the mental or emotional health of the supervisee or themselves. In such situations an empathic stance in relation to the supervisee and themselves is important alongside the consideration of the clinical material.

The focus of the organisation can also have an impact on the therapeutic and supervisory work. For example, a therapist at a 'counselling service in the United Kingdom Police Service' (Towler, 1999:p.177) described in supervision a patient, a police officer, who 'needed to keep strong' and the therapist frequently spoke of needing to 'get it right' (p.192). Both attitudes reflected aspects of the organisational police culture. In training organisations, supervision is impacted on by the training culture and requirements (see Chapter 7). It is therefore important to be aware of the organisational culture in which the supervision is taking place and its impact on the work.

Systems theory and the concept of the clinical rhombus are ways to understand the impact of organisational dynamics, but what is important for supervisors to be aware of is that a change in one part of the organisational system will change another aspect of it, which will be felt within and through the supervisory relationship. The challenge for a supervisor is exploring with their supervisees how organisational issues and changes might interrelate with, and impact on, the patient's material.

Group supervision

Supervision is often provided in groups and these have their own specific dynamics which are important to consider. Bernard & Goodyear (1998) point out that supervision groups 'minimises supervisee dependence', 'provide opportunities for vicarious learning', 'provide exposure to a broader range of clients', and 'provide a greater quantity and diversity of feedback to the supervisee' (pp.112–113). They also provide greater opportunities for developing clinical techniques and gives the supervisor 'a more comprehensive picture of the supervisee' (p.113) along with the support of others (McWilliams, 2021:p.107). However, the 'group format may not give supervisees with heavy caseloads the time they need' (Bernard & Goodyear, 1998:pp.114–115), there may be different learning needs due to different supervisory skills and some group phenomena may impede learning especially if there is a dominant group member.

Group supervision also presents the supervisor with the overlapping relational dynamics of the clinical work and the dynamics of the group and awareness of both of these are important in order to contain and keep the group focused as a supervision work group (Bion, 1989). The first meeting of a supervision group (online or in person) brings into the mix complex unconscious processes and transference and countertransference issues between the group members. For the group to develop into an effective work group a level of trust and group cohesiveness needs to develop and the supervisor needs to manage the group dynamics and issues of envy, shame, rivalry and familial dynamics if they arise (Driver, 2002b). In order to achieve a functioning work group in which the members are predominantly supportive of each other a supervisor needs to provide a group environment that is 'contained, focused on clinical work and clinical development and where anxieties are not too overwhelming and trust and intimacy can develop' (Driver, 2002b: p.86) between each member of the group and with the supervisor. In addition, a supervisor needs to encourage a supervisory alliance between the supervisees that is exploratory so that the group supervision 'can provide a reflective and supportive milieu and become a rich and valuable tool in the development of clinical work, supervisee development and good clinical practice' (Driver, 2002b:p.86).

It is also important to be aware of factors that might inhibit the supervisory alliance within a group. When supervisees in a group have different levels of experience the less experienced can feel intimidated by the more experienced. There may be envy and rivalries between members of the group, battles for authority and time and defences and anxieties about exposure. All of which can get in the way of open exploration of the patient material. However, the group is a supervision group and not a therapy group, so keeping the focus on the patient is important. However, sometimes group issues may need to be addressed if they are getting in the way of the supervision process, but, normally, group issues relate to supervisory issues. These may be pragmatic such as rivalries over time allocation but often group issues relate to parallel process dynamics emanating from the patient.

Group supervision therefore provides the supervisor with a rich resource in relation to the patient material and the clinical work because often the group dynamics relate to unconscious communication, identifications and projections from the patient material. For example, when a supervisee presented a patient whose parents were academics, two members of the group started talking about theory (became academics) whereas the supervisee who presented felt inferior and misunderstood; a dynamic that paralleled the patient's issues. It was through the exploratory processes within, and by, the group in relation to these identifications that the supervisees understood more about the patient.

The strength of group supervision is that it provides a wider forum for the exploration of clinical work. Firstly, in groups 'a third party is always present to witness the interaction of any dyad. This presence of an observing third is a source of enormous potential for understanding the complex relational themes that unfold in any supervisory situation' (Frawley-O'Dea and Sarnat, 2001:p.201). Secondly, group supervision 'provides the possibility for a freer-flowing associative process than does individual supervision' and 'just as two heads are often better than one, so multiple heads can be better still if their emotional and cognitive synergies can be effectively channelled' (p.201). In addition, group supervision provides a multi-person resource in terms of support, sharing thoughts and feelings, exploring unconscious identifications and parallel process. However, it is also important that the supervisor engages in internal reflection about their own countertransference in order to understand the dynamics of the group in relation to the work with the patient (Driver, 2002b:p.95). It is the supervisory relationships within a group that holds the potential for a rich and deep exploration of the patient material.

Peer supervision

For practical reasons as well as a means of overcoming the isolation of therapeutic work and the requirements of continuing professional development (CPD) peer supervision is often chosen by qualified practitioners. The advantage of peer supervision is that it enables ongoing reflection of clinical work and transference and countertransference and is a forum in which new information and ideas can be shared and explored. There is usually no designated role of supervisee or supervisor because each person takes a turn in either role. In addition, peer supervision can offer a supportive environment in which the isolation of therapeutic work and potential burn-out can be avoided (Bernard and Goodyear, 1998: p. 127) and normally no payment is involved. However, the disadvantages are that challenging each other can be difficult and avoided, a member of the group may become dominant, collusion and defences may arise against anything negative in order to maintain a good feeling in the group or the group collapses into a social group.

In order to mitigate some of these problems, a range of ground rules have been proposed by a number of writers in relation to peer-group supervision (Bernard and Goodyear, 1998; Hawkins and Shohet, 2002; Kassan, 2010). The consensus is that a contract amongst members of the peer group is helpful in terms of how the group time is allocated and who leads the group. Bernard and Goodyear (1998) comment that in peer groups 'ignoring the issue of leadership gives rise to competitiveness' and that the best approach is a rotation of the 'leadership role with one person directing each meeting' (p.128). Other issues to consider include agreeing who is presenting at each meeting, ensuring this is rotated equally, agreeing an ongoing commitment to the group and clarifying the expectations of the group (Hawkins and Shohet, 2002). Bernard and Goodyear (1998) also suggest that 'a process observer be appointed (different from either the presenter or the designated leader)' (p.128). Their role is to give feedback at the 'end of the supervision meeting about the group process, the group's ability to stay task focused' (p.128) and offer relevant reflections in relation to the supervisory process. Peer supervision is an option that many qualified practitioners choose and it has clear advantages but clarity about how such a group runs will alleviate some of the pitfalls.

Difference and diversity in supervision

A major factor to consider in supervision are issues of gender, sexuality, race, class, culture, disability, language, generational difference and other aspects of difference and diversity. Both supervisors and supervisees bring to the supervisory relationship their 'acculturated self' (Knorpel and Cockersell, 2024) in terms of their personal and cultural identity, life view and attitudes, all of which affects their attitude and understanding of the patient material and each other.

When training to be psychoanalysts and psychotherapists the theory we are presented with is mostly meta-psychology in relation to the structure and functioning of the mind/psyche. Exploring issues of difference and diversity requires a much broader way of thinking and understanding and an awareness of the intersectional vectors (Crenshaw, 1989), which form 'a person's social and political identity … *and* …combine to create different modes of discrimination and privilege' (Agoro, 2024:p.40). As supervisors we have a responsibility to model ways of exploring issues of difference and diversity in relation to patients and supervisees. However, this is no easy task as often a supervisee or supervisor may find it hard to address issues of difference and diversity because they touch on areas of their own personal identity or feelings of shame, embarrassment or, perhaps, power. Lago and Thompson (1997) identified how often a patient, therapist/supervisee and supervisor will operate from a proxy or false self 'in order to protect their real self' (p.124) and fit in. As a result direct communication and real understanding of the supervisee/therapist or patient fails to occur. It is therefore important for supervisors 'to learn from our supervisees about such issues as they pertain to them individually' (McWilliams, 2021:p.181) through conversations with them.

To truly address issues of difference and diversity in supervision requires the supervisor to be aware or their own assumptions and prejudices and be willing to step into the unknown to discover the real issues that are being presented by the patient and/or therapist/ supervisee. Lago and Thompson (1997) cite Atkinson et al. (1983) who advocates that supervisors need 'to have some general knowledge about – the formation of racial and cultural identities, cultural norms, racial conflicts' (p.122) and a willingness to address these issues. However, the challenge for supervisors (and therapists) is that we mostly don't know, and can't know, all the elements related to difference and diversity for an individual. The important factor is a willingness and humility to accept not knowing and for the supervisor to explore, discover, and understand, with the supervisee, what the patient or supervisee's experience has been and how it has affected them. Watkins and Hook (2016) refer to such a process as culturally humble psychoanalytic supervision. They comment that 'realizing cultural humility via supervisory interaction involves the opening of a supervisor-supervisee third space whereby cultural meanings and experiences *and difference and diversity* [1] are welcomed and can be explored, examined, and experienced anew' (p.487). By exploring in this way the supervisor generates 'a prototype for the supervisee/patient's own creation of a cultural third' (p.487).

The importance of humility as a mindset in supervision is significant because it identifies the need for the supervisor (or supervisee) to step down from the potential arrogance of knowing, or being in a position of power, to a place of openness to not knowing and facing the challenge of what might be uncomfortable realities and dynamics. As Watkins and Hook (2016) go on to comment,

culturally humble psychoanalytic supervision rests on a foundation of four components: (a) cultural self-awareness, (b) cultural awareness of the other, (c) a culturally sensitive supervisory alliance, and (d) culturally sensitive intervention strategies and techniques.

(p.498)

Acknowledging that the other, the supervisee or the patient, might know and understand more about a particular issue than the supervisor underpins supervisory humility especially in relation to diversity and difference. Addressing issues relating to difference and diversity is vital and requires humility and a secure base so as to be 'free to explore … and engage with difference' (Power, 2016:p.36).

For example, an Afro-Caribbean supervisee, Jocelyn, who I was supervising online, worked as a therapist seeing patients in person in an Afro-Caribbean community project. In talking about one patient she frequently interspersed her presentation with the phrase "you know". However, I felt I "didn't know" what she or the patient meant. I felt embarrassed to admit this to myself, but realised I needed to in order to understand the patient's life, inner world and the dynamics of the therapy. I was aware that the patient and Jocelyn seemed to identify with each other and maybe did "know" what the other was talking about, whereas I, as a white person, was outside of it. Also, working with Jocelyn online amplified my feeling of being outside of Jocelyn's and the patient's world. I said to Jocelyn that I felt she and the patient were in the same world and understood each other but that I, as a white person, and not part of the project, was outside of it and found it hard to understand what she seemed to "know". I asked Jocelyn to tell me more about what she knew and how she understood the patient. Jocelyn replied that she sort of "knew" what the family dynamics were for her patient because they were both from the same Afro-Caribbean country and that in the area in which they lived there was a sort of prohibition about talking openly to white people and someone like me. This conversation in relation to the supervisory dynamic and context opened up further understanding about the cultural dynamics for the patient, issues around belonging and the patient's struggles to separate from her family.

Supervisory humility, being open with the supervisee, conversation and exploration are all ways of opening up and understanding issues of difference and diversity. This requires an attitude of mind in the supervisor that must overcome assumptions, prejudice, arrogance and power and attune to the challenges and issues that patients and supervisees bring in relation to their own experience and their own identity and reality. An ability to explore issues of difference and diversity also increases the level of trust and openness between supervisee and supervisor and deepens the supervisory alliance.

Mistakes in supervision

Supervisee shame and/or a desire to do well and get positive feedback from the supervisor often inhibits a supervisee from talking about mistakes. But mistakes are often important pieces of information because they sometimes hold meaning in relation to the patient. Nagell et al., (2014) comment, 'mistakes should be used as a source of understanding unconscious processes' (p.576). To enable a supervisee to talk about their mistakes requires trust in the supervisory alliance that the supervisor will be open to hearing about them. Mistakes might include a supervisee forgetting things in supervision or being unable to remembers parts of the session with the patient when presenting, which might resonate with the patient's defences about issues they don't want to consciously think about. Or they could be an enactment such as forgetting a session which might reflect the patient's experience of a disorganised attachment with their parents. Mistakes can, therefore, hold symbolic significance and reflect unconscious issues and projections in relation to the patient. Casement (2002) has written extensively about mistakes in practice and comments on the inevitability of them and how, in supervision, they can turn into a means for growth for the therapist as well as the patient (Casement, 2002).

Sometimes, however, mistakes are more serious and a supervisor needs to be alert to when mistakes become boundary violations or ethical issues (see also Chapter 8). The task for the supervisor is to determine whether a mistake is symbolic and informative about the work with the patient or reflects an ethical or competence issue in relation to the supervisee.

Endings in supervision

Endings in supervision occur for a variety of reasons, such as organisational changes, training requirements or the changing needs of a practitioner. In fact, changing supervisor from time to time is helpful and important as it provides a practitioner with different perspectives and ways of thinking and working. Zachrisson (2011) considers that, in training, candidates should have 'two or three supervisors to provide them with more than one model of thinking, and more than one analytic dialect, from which to develop their own psychoanalytic language and their own analytic identity' (p.951). Mander (2002b) raises the important question of whether there is an optimal length of time for a supervisory contract. She comments that as long as supervision remains a process of discovery through a 'togetherness of thinking' and exploration it is valuable but 'when it becomes stale, monotonous, boring and repetitive it is time to leave' (Mander, 2002b:p.141) and end the supervisory relationship. It is also important to reflect on the impact of who ends the supervisory relationship; supervisor, supervisee or the organisational setting. Mander comments that 'when the ending is initiated by one of the supervisory partners, and not mutually, there may remain an air of betrayal, resentment, and rejection' (2002b:p.149). It is especially challenging if a supervisor ends the supervision when there is a positive transference to them. As a supervisor it is also important to accept that 'supervisees grow and develop and may outgrow their supervisors, just as the relationship between parents and children is always liable to change over time' (Crawford, 2005: p.59).

For whatever reason, when a supervisory relationship ends the ending needs to be worked with sensitively. A decision to end supervision should normally be planned and worked towards and the supervisor needs to be alert to how issues of change and loss may get paralleled in the presentation of the supervisee or the dynamics with the patient. In addition, attention needs to be given to what arrangements the practitioner has made for further supervision and the work with the patients. A key factor for the supervisor, when a supervisee ends, are the patients and 'whether they carry on with the supervisee (but are lost to the supervisor) or finish at the same time (and are lost to both participants)' (Mander, 2002b:p.149). In one case, the patient's therapeutic journey remains unfinished for the supervisor and in the latter it remains unfinished for both supervisee and supervisor; something that needs to be acknowledged by the supervisor as a loss alongside the ending with the supervisee.

Sometimes, however supervision ends for more difficult reasons. If problems arise in the supervisory relationship, which cannot be worked through, and is inhibiting the supervisee's work with their patients, then a supervisor may need to end the supervisory relationship and enable the supervisee to find another supervisor so that the work with their patients can progress. A more challenging scenario is when there is a fitness to practice issue. In such situations a supervisor will need to take an authoritative and managerial role in relation to ending the work of the supervisee and ensure that the supervisee ends their work with patients and closes their practice. Supervisory consultation for the supervisor in such a situation is both supportive and helpful in working with such difficult and challenging situations.

Final comment

The development of the supervisory relationship and the supervisory alliance enables a creative, open and exploratory relationship. This takes time and requires the supervisor to be aware of the needs and anxieties of the supervisee even though they may not be explored directly. In addition, the supervisor needs to be aware of issues of difference and diversity and the impact of the patient material and context (organisational or private practice) on the processes and dynamics of supervision. However, the dynamics of supervision are never static, they change over time and change with every new patient brought and every session presented. The supervisory relationship and alliance are the basis of in-depth supervisory work and the establishment of this in supervision enables the supervisee to internalise a reflective and reflexive capacity and work from this with their patients.

Note

1   My addition in italics.

References

Agoro, O. (2024) 'Supervision within the context of decolonisation'. Ababio, B. (ed.) *Intercultural Supervision in Therapeutic Practice*. Oxon and New York: Routledge.

Atkinson, D., Morton, G. and Sue, D.W. (1983) *Counselling American Minorities: A Cross Cultural Perspective*. Dubuque, IA: Williams C. Brown.

Bernard, J.M. and Goodyear, R.K. (1998) *Fundamentals of Clinical Supervision*. 2nd edition. London and Toronto: Allyn and Bacon.

Bion, W.R. (1989) *Experiences in Groups*. London: Routledge.

Brown, L. and Miller, M. (2002) 'The triadic intersubjective matrix in supervision. The use of disclosure to work through painful affects'. *Int. J. Psychoanal.* (83)(4):811–823.

Casement, P. (2002) *Learning from our Mistakes*. London: Routledge.

Crawford, S. (2005) 'Free association and supervision'. Driver, C. and Martin, E. (eds.) *Supervision and the Analytic Attitude*. London: Whurr.

Crenshaw, K. (1989) 'Demarginalizing the intersection of race and sex: A black feminist critique of antidiscrimination doctrine, feminist theory and antiracist politics'. *University of Chicago Legal Forum*. Vol 1989 (1). https://chicagounbound.uchicago.edu/uclf/vol1989/iss1/8/ (Accessed 11. 2. 2024).

Driver, C. (2002a) 'Internal states in the supervisory relationship'. Driver, C. and Martin, E. (eds.) *Supervising Psychotherapy: Psychoanalytic and Psychodynamic Perspectives*. London: Sage.

Driver, C. (2002b) 'The geography and topography of supervision in a group setting'. Driver, C. and Martin, E. (eds.) *Supervising Psychotherapy: Psychoanalytic and Psychodynamic Perspectives*. London: Sage.

Driver, C. (2005) 'Attachment and the supervisory alliance'. Driver, C. and Martin, E. (eds.) *Supervision and the Analytic Attitude*. London: Whurr.

Frawley-O'Dea, M.G. and Sarnat, J.E. (2001) *The Supervisory Relationship*. New York: The Guilford Press.

Hawkins, P. and Shohet, R. (2002) *Supervision in the Helping Professions*, 2nd edition. Buckingham and Philadelphia: Open University Press.

Kassan, L.D. (2010) *Peer Supervision Groups: How They Work and Why You Need One*. Northvale, NJ: Jason Aronson.

Knorpel, A. and Cockersell, P. (2024) 'Drawing attention to what is and isn't said, seen, heard, felt, and communicated in the Intercultural supervisory space'. Ababio, B. (ed.) *Intercultural Supervision in Therapeutic Practice*. Oxon and New York: Routledge.

Lago, C. and Thompson, J. (1997) 'The triangle with curved sides: sensitivity to issues of race and culture in supervision'. Shipton, G. (ed.) *Supervision of Psychotherapy and Counselling*. Maidenhead: OUP.

Langs, R. (1994) *Doing Supervision and Being Supervised*. London: Karnac Books.

Langs, R. (1997) 'The framework of supervision in psychoanalytic psychotherapy'. Martindale, B.*et al.*, (eds.) *Supervision and Its Vicissitudes*. London: Karnac Books.

Mander, G. (2002a) 'Supervision: Between control and collusion'. Driver, C. and Martin, E. (eds.) *Supervising Psychotherapy*. London: Sage Publications.

Mander, G. (2002b) 'Timing and ending in supervision'. Driver, C. and Martin, E. (eds.) *Supervising Psychotherapy*. London: Sage Publications.

McWilliams, N. (2021) *Psychoanalytic Supervision*. New York and London: The Guilford Press.

Nagell, W., Steinmetzer, L., Fissabre, U., and Spilski, J. (2014) 'Research into the relationship experience in supervision and its influence on the psychoanalytical identity formation of candidate trainees'. *Psychoanal. Inq.* (34)(6):554–583.

Power, A. (2016) 'Can supervision foster the personal cultural awareness that trainings often miss out? My aspirations as a psychotherapy supervisor'. *J. Psych. Ther.* (1)(1):35–40.

Stewart, J. (2002b) 'The container and the contained: Supervision and its organisational context'. Driver, C. and Martin, E. (eds.) *Supervising Psychotherapy*. London: Sage Publications.

Towler, J. (1999) 'Supervision in uniformed settings'. Carroll, M., and Holloway, E. (eds.) *Counselling Supervision in Context*. London and Thousand Oaks, California: Sage Publications.

Watkins, C.E. (2012) 'Moments of real relationship in psychoanalytic supervision'. *Am. J. Psychoanal.* (72)(3):251–268.

Watkins, C.E. (2014) 'The supervisory alliance: A half century of theory, practice, and research in critical perspective'. *Am. J. of Psychother.* (68)(1).

Watkins, C.E. and Hook, J. (2016) 'On a culturally humble psychoanalytic supervision perspective: Creating the cultural third'. *Psychoanal. Psychol.* (33)(3):487–517.

Zachrisson, A. (2011) 'Dynamics of psychoanalytic supervision: A heuristic model'. *Int. J. Psychoanal.* (92)(4):943–961.

Chapter 4

Unconscious processes in supervision

The dynamics of the unconscious underpins all psychoanalytic and psychodynamic work, including supervision. Theories about the structure and dynamics of the unconscious have developed considerably since Freud's and Jung's original hypotheses and whilst it is not possible to go into them all in detail here, it is helpful to give a brief overview of some key theories because they identify how a supervisor can reflect on and consider the dynamics and meanings of unconscious processes, projection, transference and countertransference in supervision.

The reflection process and parallel process

Both Searles (1955) and Ekstein and Wallerstein (1958) used their understanding of unconscious processes to identify the reflection process (Searles, 1955) and parallel process (Ekstein and Wallerstein, 1958) as significant dynamics to be understood and worked with in supervision. They realised that supervision is impacted on by the unconscious via identification, projective identification and transference emanating from the patient and also the supervisee. Experienced as feelings, images and countertransference phenomena, these undercurrents from the unconscious connect to the internal world of the patient, supervisee and supervisor when imagoes, images and affects hold a symmetrical and similar valency; a dynamic that I explore later in this chapter.

DOI: 10.4324/9781003496137-4

Searles (1955) recognised that the 'the processes at work currently in the *relationship between* patient and therapist are often reflected in the *relationship between* therapist and supervisor' (p.157). He comments that 'emotions experienced by a supervisor – including even[1] their private, "subjective" fantasy experiences and their personal feelings about the supervisee' (p.157) are often 'highly informative reflections of the relationship between therapist and patient' (p.158). He emphasises that a supervisor needs to be alert to the 'possibility that the source of their emotion may lie chiefly in the therapist-patient relationship and, basically, chiefly in the patient themselves' (p.159). However, he warns that the supervisor does need to ensure that the source of their emotion 'does not lie in their own repressed past' (p.159).

Searles considered that when a patient's anxieties, or defences against anxiety, are near to awareness they connect to comparable anxieties in the therapist. These issues are then exhibited in supervision as unconscious communications in relation to something that is going on for the patient – 'something which the therapist's own anxiety prevents them from putting their finger on and consciously describing to the supervisor' (Searles, 1955:p.172). Searles considered that there is a progression in terms of anxiety and defences against anxiety. These are most intense in the patient, less intense in the therapist and come to supervisor in a more diluted form. 'It is as if the therapist were unconsciously trying, in this fashion, to tell the supervisor what the therapeutic problem is' (p.173). Later, however, he broadens out his conceptualisation of the reflection process and considers that both negative and anxiety laden dynamics and positive elements such as fondness and pleasure (p.175) can all be carried over from the patient-therapist relationship into the therapist-supervisor one.

A similar concept was proposed by Ekstein and Wallerstein (1958), which they termed parallel process. They draw attention to how events occurring between supervisor and supervisee/therapist 'illuminates difficulties existing ... between ... therapist and patient' (p.177). Their concept of parallel process links to the fact that,

> psychotherapy is an interpersonal process and what emerges
> as the therapist's perception of the interaction and of its

meanings is a reflection not only of the presenting anxieties and psychopathological manifestations of the patient, but of the level of competence and the problems in skill and in learning of the therapist.

(p.179)

Ekstein and Wallerstein (1958) consider that beginners 'frequently seem prone to respond to those aspects of their patient's problems that highlight their own specific learning problems' (p.177). These unconscious issues are then conveyed in supervision as parallel process especially when a supervisee's internal ego-reflective capacity and level of self-awareness is less developed.

However Ekstein and Wallerstein (1958) also warn that parallel process can act in reverse because both supervisor and therapist have blind spots (see Chapter 5) and issues they unconsciously get caught up in. This is important to be aware of because just as the patient material can impact on, and be paralleled in, supervision so the supervisor's experience and approach can impact on and be paralleled in the therapeutic work with the patient. In conclusion, they comment that 'students and their supervisors will work together best if each of them have active insight, achieved frequently only after struggle, into both parallel processes' (p.196).

Unconscious communication is always present within the supervisory relationship, but Searles (1955) warns that the reflection process, or parallel process, is 'only a small proportion of events which occur in supervisory hours' (p.159). However, what Searles and Ekstein and Wallerstein identify is that the dynamics of the unconscious from the patient can be unconsciously conveyed in supervision and experienced, in a more moderated form, by the supervisor. Awareness of these dynamics can lead to a deeper understanding of the patient and their internal world.

Freud, the unconscious and supervision

To consider the dynamics, manifestations and meanings of unconscious communication in supervision, it is important to keep in mind some theoretical concepts about the unconscious. Freud's topographical model of conscious, preconscious and unconscious

(Freud, 1915), his structural frame of reference of id, ego and superego (Freud, 1923) and his concept that the unconscious contains repressed mental content provide hypotheses about the unconscious. But, more important in relation to supervision is the way that Freud differentiates between primary process, the language of the unconscious, which does not obey the rules of formal logic, and secondary process, the language of consciousness and the reality principle. His most significant contribution, based on this, are his theories about the logic and 'special characteristics of the system unconscious' (Freud, 1915:p.186). Freud (1915) described these as,

- Displacement (e.g., the way an idea's emphasis, interest or intensity is liable to be detached from it and become superimposed on to other ideas).
- Condensation (several chains of association, several ideas, may be expressed through a single idea).
- Timelessness.
- Disregard of reality and the replacement of external reality by internal reality.
- Psychic reality – memories of events, real or imagined, are not distinguished.
- The absence of contradiction.
- Absence of negation.
- Words as "things" – a symbol is treated as if it were a representation of a concrete *thing*.(Sandler et al., 1997:pp.79–81)

What Freud identifies is that unconscious primary processes are timeless and fuse, replace or superimpose affects, images and memories when there is a similar valency. We experience this through the transference, unconscious communications and identifications in the therapeutic relationship and the supervisory one and they underpin the dynamics of parallel process/reflection process within supervision. Martin (2005) points out that within the unconscious 'images tend to fuse and readily replace and symbolise each other' and 'ignore categories of space and time' (p.5). He goes to comment that, 'such dynamics can create a symmetry between seemingly diverse issues or ideas' (p.7) within the unconscious and that these can be presented 'consciously through many variations and themes' (p.13). It is only through secondary process thinking, which is 'ego driven, thinking-related and adapted to the external world' (Martin, 2005:p.5) that the dynamics and projections from the unconscious can be unravelled, understood and made conscious.

Matte-Blanco (1975) developed Freud's ideas further and identified that the unconscious is a 'discriminator and classifier' (Rayner and Tuckett, 1988:p.18) and, through generalisation, 'treats an individual thing (person, object, concept) as if it were a member or element of a set or class which contains other members' (p.38). This is very pertinent to our work as supervisors. So, for example, 'a man is an element in the class of men' (p.38), which means that unconsciously issues could get generalised from one man to all men. Matte-Blanco (1975) also proposes the logic of asymmetry as belonging to consciousness and symmetry to the unconscious and that unconscious symmetrical logic leads to generalisations because all things that are of a similar valency are treated as the same and are generalised into a set of feelings or complexes of common elements. As a result of symmetrical logic an experience of an aggressive mother could unconsciously be generalised into a set of mothers with the result that all mothers would be deemed aggressive. In supervision this has serious implications if the therapist or supervisor unconsciously identifies with the symmetrical logic of the patient's unconscious. This would result in them being blind to the issues that they are caught up in. One of the challenges of supervision therefore is that until thinking, conscious awareness and asymmetry occur, both supervisee and supervisor can be symmetrically and unconsciously identified with the patient's internal and unconscious perceptions.

Ego and superego and supervision

Another key area stemming from Freud's (1923) theories is that of the ego and superego, both of which are important to consider in relation to the dynamics of supervision. Key to supervisory work is an observing ego (Greenson, 1981), the capacity to use the reflective function (Fonagy, 2001) and the development a meta-position from which to consider the issues being brought into supervision. But supervision and the supervisor can generate anxiety and regression in the supervisee, especially beginners, and as Pally points out 'a person who grew up being criticized all the time will tend to "hear" criticism in the comments of others, even when no criticism occurs' (Pally, 2007:p.865). As a result, the supervisee may feel persecuted by their persecutory superego and feel 'internally attacked' (Driver, 2023:p.6) and unable to think or reflect.

When the superego acts as a censor it determines 'what can be consciously thought in order to manage anxiety and inhibit unwanted thoughts and affects entering consciousness' (Driver, 2023:p.1). It also focuses on 'oughts, shoulds and should nots' (p.5), which inhibits reflection and exploration. As Britton (2003) comments, *'self-observation is an ego function and not a superego function*. The ego observes itself in a realistic light, the superego in a moral light' (p.72). It is therefore important for a supervisor to be aware of the impact of the superego within the patient, supervisee or themselves. 'When we find ourselves operating from a rigid superego, or from a position of "right" or "wrong", it is important to ask ourselves what this belongs to and whether we are getting caught up in our own superego dynamics or persecutory anxieties' (Driver, 2023:p 9) or whether this belongs to the patient or supervisee.

A harsh, persecutory or censorious superego will result in splitting and restrict, or inhibit, ego based reflection and exploration in supervision. In contrast a benign superego not only 'spurs and inspires the clinician to meet the demands of a training and the profession' (Driver, 2019:p.167) it also links both supervisor and supervisee to the values and ethical principles underpinning clinical work and the profession. The superego can, therefore, be a censor and a persecutor, but in its benign form it is a protector of clinical values and principles.

The container-contained and Bion

Bion's concept of the container/contained (Bion, 1970), his theory of thinking and reverie (Bion, 1967), his principles of mental functioning and his ideas about learning from experience (Bion, 1962) are all important in relation to the dynamics of supervision.

Supervision is a container, but it is also a process and Bion's
(1970) ideas in relation to the concept of the container-contained
reflect this. Ogden comments (2004a)

> in Bion's hands, the word "container"—with its benign con-
> notations of a stable, sturdy delineating function—becomes a
> word that denotes the full spectrum of ways of processing
> experience from the most destructive and deadening to the
> most creative and growth-promoting.
>
> (p.1349)

In supervision this requires the supervisor to actively engage with
both content and process and be open to thinking the unthinkable.
Ungar and Ahumada (2001) comment, 'when emotional containment is adequately handled, the supervision helps the understanding and development of the supervisee's use of his/her own
personality as a treatment instrument' (p.71). For this to occur the
supervisors' facilitative attitude is potentially transformational.

But what the supervisee presents and what the supervisor
experiences is not just about the words spoken, it is also about the
supervisee's representations of the patient material because 'the
supervisee will always give the supervisor something of the experience of the patient work, provided the supervisor is receptive and
able to understand their perceptions' (Yorke, 2005:p.35). The
supervisor's experience may include irrational experiences, phanta-
sies, unbearable states of mind or raw physiological sense data.
Bion described affects, sense data, and emotional experience, etc.,
as beta elements (Bion, 1967:p.117) and the alpha-function as the
process which 'converts sense data into alpha-elements' (p.115)
available for dreaming, consciousness and thought. Caper (1999)
developed Bion's ideas further and considered that the therapist's
use of their alpha function enables the patient's beta elements, projections and unconscious issues to be made conscious. These ideas
are equally valid for the processes of supervision. Sense data might
include physical sensations such as feeling sleepy, dizziness or a
headache or feelings such as anger, panic or anxiety, etc., or any
physical or emotional sensation that is not part of the supervisor's
or supervisee's everyday experience. When sense data remain

unprocessed in supervision it will be projected or evacuated into the supervisor or the supervisory relationship. The supervisor's alpha function is therefore necessary in order to process, consider, work with and understand the real, disturbing and sometimes visceral experiences that hearing about a patient can generate.

If a supervisor can maintain a capacity to hold and reflect on affects, sense data, emotional experiences, disturbing thoughts and dream thoughts, and use their alpha-function to consider these communications from the unconscious, this is both containing and potentially enriching. Bion (1967) commented that 'thinking is a development forced on the psyche by the pressure of thoughts and not the other way round' (p.111). Ogden (2008), commenting on Bion's work, says that it 'requires two minds to think a person's most disturbing thoughts' (p.12) and supervision provides a forum in which thoughts can be consciously shared and explored between supervisor and supervisee. A process that enables the supervisee to develop a deeper understanding of the patient and their work with the patient. The containing capacity of the mental functioning of the supervisor is vital if unconscious communication from the patient is to be processed and understood, but it is a process that requires internal and external dialogue; internal dialogue within the supervisor and external dialogue with the supervisee in order to discover and find a deeper understanding of the issues presented by the patient. In owning the affects, and entering into an internal and external dialogue, beta-elements of unprocessed experience become, through reverie, thinking and reflecting, thoughts that lead to understanding. A process representing the container-contained function of supervision.

Unconscious dynamics and supervision

Ideas based on object relations theory such as projection, projective identification, transference, countertransference and the paranoid schizoid and depressive positions (Klein, 1975, 1988) are also helpful to consider in relation to supervision. If a supervisee, or supervisor, operates from the paranoid schizoid position issues concerning the patient or the supervisee will be related to in a one-sided way. For example, when a patient talks about their 'terrible' partner the supervisee might talk about the partner in supervision in an equivalent way by, say, demonising the partner. Such a perspective may indicate splitting based on paranoid-schizoid thinking and the symmetrical logic that Matte-Blanco refers to. If the supervisor colludes with this split alternative perspectives cannot be reached. However, if the supervisor can enable a shift in thinking whereby the perspective of the patient and the partner can be considered in an open and reflective way a link to a deeper understanding of the patient and their patterns of relating, based on the depressive position, can be achieved.

All our theories about the unconscious provide potential insight into the operation of the unconscious in supervision. Attachment theory identifies how the internal working models (Holmes, 1993) and attachment patterns (Driver, 2005; Power, 2014) affect patient, supervisee and possibly also the supervisor in terms of how they relate to each other. Jung saw the unconscious as being personal, collective (common to all humanity) and purposeful and he frequently used metaphors to describe unconscious and intra- and inter-relational dynamics. In particular, he made use of the alchemical metaphor (Jung, 1946) to consider the dynamics of the transference and the therapeutic relationship, which Allphin (2005) applied to the supervisory one. This process describes how the dynamics of the opposites (Jung, 1916/57), such as attraction or conflict, are a fundamental dynamic of the psyche which, if they are identified and worked through, can create a new perspective or way of thinking. Jung considered 'that effective psychological treatment' (Jung, 1929:para.163) requires the unconscious of the patient to impact on and inform the therapist. Ideas that are equally applicable to the dynamics of supervision.

The impact of the context of the clinical and/or supervisory work is also a factor to consider. Kernberg (2010) identifies the prevalence of paranoid fears in authoritarian organisations (p.610) and that such fears can be activated in training settings especially when assessments are required. In addition, working in organisations can generate a range of feelings including frustration, envy, rivalry, fear and anxiety all of which can creep into the supervisory relationship and the dynamics of supervision. This is where a supervisor needs to be aware of the conscious and unconscious impact of the setting on both supervisee(s) and supervisor so as to identify the unconscious issues linked to the organisation as well as any parallel process in relation to the patient material.

Intersubjectivity and inter-relational dynamics in supervision

The theories of our profession all provide a rich spectrum from which to understand the unconscious and internal world. The purpose of this understanding is in order to process and understand the patient, the experience of being with the patient and the experience with the supervisee. It is through the inter-personal and intra-psychic dynamics of the overlapping relationship of patient, supervisee and supervisor that experiences, conscious and unconscious, are shared. These ideas relate to the concept of the therapeutic fenceless field (Fordham, 1995), Racker's (1982) theories about transference and concordant or complimentary counter-transference[2] and the intersubjectivity of therapeutic relationships (Ogden, 1999, 2004b). Based on a Winnicottian perspective Ogden (2004b) examines how he reflects on, and is receptive to, an inter-subjective third space and how superseding the third occurs through recognition and reappropriation of 'the (transformed) individual subjectivities of the participants' (p.169). Through this process each participant becomes aware of what belongs to them and what belongs to the other. Dynamics that are at play in the supervisory relationship.

Supervision is a complex relationship that is consciously and unconsciously affected by all aspects of the clinical rhombus (Ekstein and Wallerstein, 1958) and in order to determine the impact of these factors requires a supervisor to develop what Hawkins and Shohet (2002) describe as an helicopter ability that can 'switch focus' (p.44) between, and on to, the various aspects of supervision. A supervisor therefore needs to develop this capacity and find a meta-perspective, or fifth perspective, which can hover, rotate and consider the input and effect of all the various parameters that consciously and unconsciously impact on supervision. Identifying and reflecting on these various dynamics (see Chapters 1 and 6) can begin to open up awareness and understanding of what is unconsciously being communicated and carried into supervision and generate a greater understanding of the patient material.

Examples in practice

Individual supervision

Considering unconscious processes in supervision requires a supervisor to maintain a reflective analytic attitude and reverie in relation to their own internal processes and the dynamics and processes occurring between them and their supervisee(s). In this way a supervisor can begin their own internal dialogue and mind-making activities in relation to countertransference affects, thoughts, feelings and imaginings in relation to the patient and the session material because when a supervisee presents 'there remains material not part of the report or the observable session, psychic material that only psychic processes will reveal' (Yorke, 2005:p.34). Yorke goes on to comment that when 'memories and desires are evoked in supervision, they are part of the supervision and should be regarded as valid material' (p.38). Such dynamics are all part of the way in which unconscious identifications and unconscious communications can be experienced within the relational activity of supervision which the following examples illustrate.

A supervisee, Amy, new to clinical work, began seeing a female patient, Sarah. Sarah, aged 23, was an only child and lived with her parents. She had just started her first job as a teacher. Sarah described her parents as caring but strict and that she was always anxious because her Dad was critical if she didn't do well. She also described being anxious in her new job because she feared she was not doing well. In supervision, Amy presented what Sarah had told her but found it hard to talk about what she had said and looked embarrassed and flustered when I, her supervisor, asked her to say more. I felt frustrated because any exploration was closed down by Amy's lack of response and I felt critical of Amy's apparent lack of clinical skills and engagement with the patient. I was tempted to make a critical comment to Amy about this.

The power of my feelings caused me to reflect on what they might unconsciously connect to. I sensed that we (Sarah, Amy and myself as supervisor) were all caught in a parallel process of critical figures which, through the dynamics of displacement, condensation and timelessness, settled onto any figure that the unconscious experienced as parental or paternal. I decided that the best response in this situation was to comment on how powerful the fear of criticism was and empathically engage with Amy about Sarah's anxieties stemming from her critical father. This enabled Amy to begin to consider, and reflect on, the power of Sarah's superego and its links to Sarah's internalised critical parent.

Group supervision

Kernberg (2010) writes that 'in a group situation, there is an opportunity to examine the clinical aspects of a case from many different perspectives, thereby providing a richness and diversity of understanding that does not privilege any one line of thought over another' (p.612). This is because in a group, unconscious identifications by the group members may connect to aspects of the patient material and may be enactments of parallel process in relation to the patient's internal world. Remaining aware of both the patient material and possible parallel process dynamics can enable the group to explore the issues in a deeper way and identify what is being unconsciously communicated by the patient.

In a supervision group of three, comprising two female (Nazrin and Claire) and one male supervisee (Iain), Iain presented two sessions with his patient, a young woman who was very depressed. Whilst Iain was talking about the patient I found myself thinking about my forthcoming holiday and getting away from it all. I rapidly brought myself back from my imaginings and began to wonder what I was escaping from and what this might connect to. At the same time I was aware that Nazrin had begun to ask Iain lots of questions and Iain sounded quite irritated. Claire hadn't said a word and just sat quietly watching the other two. Although I did not yet understand what the responses to Iain's presentation were about I felt that they might connect to the patient. I commented to the group that something seemed to have been stirred up by the patient's material and that I wondered what they were feeling. Iain said he felt very angry and irritated by the patient and her passivity. Nazrin commented that her questions to Iain were an attempt to find out more about the patient so as to understand her better. I reflected that Claire hadn't said anything and wondered how she felt. Claire commented that she had felt afraid to comment.

Internally I reflected on the various responses; Claire's fear, Iain's anger and irritation, Nazrin's feisty questioning and my fantasy escape. There was clearly something that was hard to face which stirred up different feelings. I commented to the group on our various responses to the patient material and said that I wondered whether we were all picking up aspects of the patient's internal world and parental imagoes. Iain commented that the relationship of the patient's parents sounded quite volatile but that he did not know much more because the patient found it hard to speak about her family. I commented that perhaps there was something the patient was fearful of talking about or wanted to escape from but that it was not yet clear what that was. My comment enabled further reflection by the group members. Claire said that her fear had made it hard to say anything, especially when Iain had sounded irritated by Nazrin's questions, and that she wondered if the patient was fearful too. Iain reflected that he often found the patient irritating but had found it hard to admit this because he felt he wasn't supposed to feel like that towards a patient. Nazrin commented that she had felt annoyed at Iain and was questioning to find out more. I commented that all feelings needed to be considered because some may reflect an identification with the patient's feelings or her experience.

I felt the group were identifying with different aspects of the patient's internal world and experience of her parents. Rather than comment on this directly I asked the group to reflect on their feelings and consider what the patient might be struggling with. Nazrin said she wondered about her questioning stance and Iain's irritation and whether that reflected something in relation to the patient's parents. Iain commented that this might be true and wondered if his wish to overlook his feelings might also relate to that. Claire said that she wondered if the patient felt intimidated and frightened by her parents because that was certainly what she had felt when Nazrin and Iain were talking. After further discussion, Iain said he felt there was something about the patient's background that he didn't know about or understand and wondered if the patient was afraid to talk about it. He also wondered whether his irritation was a complementary countertransference (Racker, 1982) linked to the patient's father. The supervision ended with us all being in a state of not knowing, but aware that a range of strong feelings had been stirred up. It was with this awareness that Iain saw his patient for the next session.

When Iain presented again he commented that during the session with this patient he had been more aware of his countertransference and able to reflect on it. He had also been aware of a sense of anxiety when the patient was talking about her childhood and he had commented on this to her. This had led to the patient talking about her fear of her father and his violent outbursts. In supervision, the group was able to reflect on their previous experience of Iain's presentation of this patient and how their individual responses had resonated with aspects of the patient's internal world and been paralleled in the group. Through processes of transference and projection each member of the group had identified with an aspect of the patient. Claire with the patient's fear and Iain, through his angry and irritated countertransference, with the patient's internalised aggressive father. Nazrin seemed to have identified with a feisty, and maybe volatile, mother and I, in my fantasy, had wanted to escape the uncomfortable feelings and dynamics. All of which seemed to reflect aspect of the patient's internal world.

Group dynamics, the personalities of the supervision group members and the projections carried into the group by the patient material can set up unconscious symmetrical identifications with aspects of a patient's unconscious and patterns of relating. When this occurs it provides a rich source of information if the supervisor and the supervisees are able to reflect and think about their feelings and responses. This can sometimes be difficult because shame, envy or superego dynamics get in the way, which it nearly did with Iain and his shame at feeling irritated by the patient. Group dynamics in supervision are not always about parallel process but it is important for the supervisor to be open to the possibility. This means being open to thinking and reflecting on everything that occurs in the group, including their own internal phantasies/fantasies, and consider and explore whether they might be connected to aspects of the patient's history, internal world and unconscious dynamics.

Final comment

This chapter can only give a very brief summary and overview of ideas and theories about the dynamic properties of the unconscious. There are differences in the theories and their underlying epistemologies, but there are also common themes. They all identify the importance of unconscious communication and all identify that the unconscious coalesces themes and affects when they hold a similar valency. The theories also serve to remind us of the ever-present power of the unconscious in therapy and supervision. We may experience the unconscious slightly differently when working online rather than in person but it is still present in the way we react, feel and perceive what we see and hear. The way a supervisee speaks, what they omit and what they attach emotion to all have unconscious resonances and meaning. In addition, the way a supervisee uses the supervision session, or online facilities, all hold unconscious communications, which may be benign (e.g., sometimes being late is unavoidable) or may have meaning in relation to patient or supervisee issues.

The way we, as a supervisor, feel or react all connect to the unconscious and may parallel issues about the patient. In addition, the dynamics of the clinical rhombus generates an interactive matrix of both conscious and unconscious elements that need to be understood. Having a theoretical underpinning from which to consider the dynamics of supervision enables a supervisor to begin to think about what, and how, unconscious issues are communicated and their impact and meaning. It takes time for a supervisor to develop the capacity to reflect on, and make use of, unconscious processes in supervision, but it is important for a supervisor to be aware of the dynamic impact of unconscious communication so as to consider the unconscious and its manifestations in the supervisory relationship. The challenge for the supervisor, together with the supervisee, is to unravel, identify and understand the meaning of the unconscious communication in relation to the patient.

Notes

1 In some quotes I have replaced the word he or his with the word their so that it is not gender specific.
2 Racker (1982) coined the term complementary countertransference to refer to an identification with internal objects of the patient and concordant countertransference to an identification with the internal world and 'psychological contents' of the patient (p.135).

References

Allphin, C. (2005) 'Supervision as an alchemical process'. Driver, C., and Martin, E. (eds.) *Supervision and the Analytic Attitude*. London: Whurr.

Bion, W.R. (1962) *Learning from Experience*. London: Heinemann.

Bion, W.R. (1967) *Second Thoughts*. New York: Aronson.

Bion, W.R. (1970) *Attention and Interpretation*. London: Tavistock Publications Ltd.

Britton, R. (2003) *Sex, Death, and the Superego*. London: Karnac.

Caper, R. (1999) *A Mind of One's Own*. London and New York: Routledge.

Driver, C. (2005) 'Attachment and the supervisory alliance'. Driver, C., and Martin, E. (eds.) *Supervision and the Analytic Attitude*. London: Whurr.

Driver, C. (2019) 'The superego as a significant factor in clinical training'. Harding, C. (ed.) *Dissecting the Superego*. London: Routledge.

Driver, C. (2023) 'The superego in supervision. Censor, persecutor or protector'. *Psychodynamic Practice*. https://doi.org/10.1080/14753634.2023.2282721.

Ekstein, R., & Wallerstein, R.S. (1958) *The Teaching and Learning of Psychotherapy*. Madison Connecticut: International Universities Press, Inc.

Fonagy, P. (2001) *Attachment Theory and Psychoanalysis*. New York: Other Press.

Fordham, M. (1995) *Freud, Jung, Klein. The Fenceless Field*. Hobdell, R. (ed.) London: Routledge.

Freud, S. (1915) *The Unconscious. SE* XIV. London: Hogarth Press.

Freud, S. (1923) 'The Ego and the Id'. *The Ego and the Id and Other Works. SE* XIX. London. Hogarth Press.

Greenson, R.R. (1981) *The Technique and Practice of Psychoanalysis*. London: Hogarth Press.

Hawkins, P. & Shohet, R. (2002) *Supervision in the Helping Professions*, 2nd edition. Buckingham and Philadelphia: Open University Press.

Holmes, J. (1993) *John Bowlby and Attachment Theory*. East Sussex and New York: Brunner-Routledge.

Jung, C.G. (1916/57) 'The transcendent function'. *Structure and Dynamics of the Psyche, CW* 8. London: Routledge. 1991.

Jung, C.G. (1929) 'Problems of modern psychotherapy'. *The Practice of Psychotherapy, CW* 16. (London and Henley: Routledge & Kegan Paul). 1981.

Jung, C.G. (1946) 'The psychology of the transference'. *The Practice of Psychotherapy, CW16*. London and Henley: Routledge & Kegan Paul. 1981.

Kernberg, O.F. (2010) 'Psychoanalytic supervision: The supervisor's tasks'. *Psychoanal. Q.* (79) (3):603–627.

Klein, M. (1975) *Envy and Gratitude*. London: The Hogarth Press.

Klein, M. (1988) *Love, Guilt and Reparation*. London: Virago Press.

Martin, E. (2005) 'The unconscious in supervision'. Driver, C., and Martin, E. (eds.) *Supervision and the Analytic Attitude*. London: Whurr.

Matte-Blanco, I. (1975) *The Unconscious as Infinite Sets*. London: Karnac Books. 1998.

Ogden, T.H. (1999) *Reverie and Interpretation*. London: Karnac Books.

Ogden, T.H. (2004a) 'On holding and containing, being and dreaming'. *International Journal of Psychoanalysis* (85):1349–1364.

Ogden, T. (2004b) 'The analytic third: the implications for psychoanalytic theory and technique'. *Psychoanal. Quart.* LXXIII.

Ogden, T.H. (2008) 'Bion's four principles of mental functioning'. *fort da* (14) (2):11–35. Reprinted from Ogden. T.H. (2008) *Rediscovering Psychoanalysis: Thinking and Dreaming, Learning and Forgetting*. London: New Library of Psychoanalysis. Routledge.

Pally, R. (2007) 'The Predicting Brain'. *International Journal of Psychoanalysis* (88):861–881.

Power, A. (2014) 'Impasse in Supervision—Looking Back and Thinking Again'. *Attach: New Dir. Rel. Psychoanal. Psychother.* (8) (2):154–171.

Racker, H. (1982) *Transference and Countertransference*. London: Maresfield Library, Karnac.

Rayner, E., & Tuckett, D. (1988) 'An Introduction to Matte-Blanco's reformulation of the Freudian unconscious and his conceptualization of the internal world'. Matte-Blanco, I. (ed.) *Thinking, Feeling, and Being*. London: Routledge.

Sandler, J., Holder, A., Dare, C., and Dreher, A.U. (1997) *Freud's Models of the Mind*. London: Karnac Books.

Searles, H.F. (1955) 'The informational value of the supervisor's emotional experiences'. Searles, H.F. (1986) *Collected Papers on Schizophrenia and Related Subjects*. London: Maresfield Library.

Ungar, V., and Ahumada, L. (2001). 'Supervision. A Container-Contained Approach.' *Int. J. Psychoanal.* (82) (1):71–81.

Yorke, V. (2005) 'Bion's 'vertex' as a supervisory object'. Driver, C., and Martin, E. (eds.) *Supervision and the Analytic Attitude*. London: Whurr.

Chapter 5

Learning and development in supervision

A key role for a supervisor is to enable the supervisee to learn and develop the skills, competencies and attributes involved in being an effective psychoanalytic or psychodynamic practitioner, something that is a lifelong process because learning in supervision is a multi-faceted process, not a straightforward linear one. It requires both cognitive learning as well as emotional, affective and reflective learning in order to process what is heard and experienced with patients. Piaget (1958), and later Szecsödy (1990, 1997), point out that the learning process requires both assimilative learning, the accumulation of new knowledge and information, and accommodative learning, which enables the 'modification of existing cognitive (and emotional) schemata … by restructuring previously held knowledge, points of view and theory' (Szecsödy, 1997:p.109). Learning to become a clinician therefore requires shifts in patterns of perception and 'internal objects' (Martin, 2002a) and 'relearning in relation to cognitive, affective and behavioural experience' (Watkins and Scaturo, 2014:p.619). Effective supervision changes the perception of the supervisee and the supervisor in relation to the patient.

Learning in supervision is therefore not just about theory but about learning how to process the experience with the patient in order to understand the patient. It involves the integration of theory and practice and the development of the capacity to think, reflect and acquire a 'third position', or observing ego, and reflective function that can learn from, and through, experience. A supervisor therefore needs to enable the supervisee to listen and decode what they hear and experience with the patient in terms of

DOI: 10.4324/9781003496137-5

their thoughts, feelings, transference and countertransference affects and, explore, reflect, discuss, imagine and hypothesise with the supervisee so as to enable them to understand the patient's transference issues, patterns of relating and inner world. In addition, learning in supervision is about developing the supervisee's clinical skills so that they become an effective clinician.

Learning in supervision

Psychoanalytic and psychodynamic supervision needs to be grounded in its theoretical foundations, whatever that orientation might be, but supervisors also need to be 'informed by educational psychology and theories of learning and instruction' (Watkins, 2013: p.469) and be aware of the different learning styles and learning needs of their supervisees. Kolb (1984, 2015) and Kolb and Kolb (2005) identified that learning occurs through a cycle of experience, reflection, thought and the testing of the ideas that emerge. Supervision utilises this learning cycle when it enables exploration of the supervisee's experience of the patient, reflection and thinking about the patient and their internal world and exploration into ways of working with the patient.

Learning in supervision has been examined in detail by Watkins and Scaturo (2014). They identify that learning in supervision needs to occur through three domains: affective learning, cognitive learning and behavioural learning (p.621) in which,

- affective emotional learning relates to identification 'of the learner's feelings, values and motives and emotional experience';
- cognitive learning to the development of an 'informational base, intellectual skills, thought processes, remembering, understanding, analysing, evaluating, creating and applying';
- behavioural learning in which the supervisee translates thought into action through practicing and role play.

(Watkins and Scaturo, 2014:pp.621–629)

They conclude that those three domains of learning are critical within supervision because 'knowledge-based (think), attitudinal-based (feel), and skills-based (do)' (p.622) processes underpin the development of learning in supervision and each overlap and feed into the other.

This is the basis of experiential learning and supervision provides a space to enable this. Experiential learning in supervision involves developing the capacity to reflect on the emotional impact of the patient, the internal world and psychological functioning of the patient and their patterns of relating. This involves shifts in awareness and understanding in the supervisee and the supervisor and being open to new perspectives in order to develop understanding about the patient and how to work effectively with them.

Learning styles

Supervisors also need to consider that individuals (supervisees) have different learning styles and 'particular ways of processing information and different preferences in learning. These do not indicate differential ability' (Bernard and Goodyear, 1998:p.36). Kolb (1984) identified a range of learning styles such as diverging, converging, assimilating and accommodating and that learning can be influenced by an individual's current or previous professional career, educational specialization, adaptive competences, personality type (Kolb and Kolb, 2005:p.6), culture and belief systems.

Typology such as thinking, feeling, intuition or sensation (Jung, 1921) or the thinking, feeling, sensing, intuition, judging, perceiving perspective of the Myers-Briggs' typology (Meyers, 1962) also identifies the different ways individuals perceive and learn. So, for example, someone who is predominantly a thinking type may find it difficult to consider feelings. Bernard and Goodyear (1998) identified that 'thinking-judging supervisors will find a trainee who makes decisions based on subjective data to be frustrating' and that 'feeling-perceiving trainees may in fact be more capable of achieving empathy with clients than their supervisors' (p.36). Typology is a factor to consider when there is a divergence of approach between supervisor and supervisee in relation to the clinical material. However, as supervisors, we need to be aware that a particular typology may become a defensive retreat from anxiety provoking material, e.g., thinking to avoid feeling, in either supervisor or supervisee, or a particular typology might be activated by the patient material.

A developmental model of learning in supervision

Supervisors also need to take into account the level of experience of a supervisee because learning in supervision is a developmental process. Stoltenberg and Delworth (1987), Szecsödy (1990, 2013), Kernberg (1996, 2006, 2007, 2010), Bernard and Goodyear (1998), Hawkins and Shohet (2002), Thomas (2005), Watkins (2013, 2016) and others identify that 'supervision is a developmentally anchored educational experience in which the supervisory relationship serves as the crucible of supervisee change' (Watkins, 2016:p.437) as they train to become a clinician. It is therefore important for supervisors to be aware of the level of experience of their supervisees and the style of supervision that may be required to enable the supervisee to become a psychoanalytic or psychodynamic practitioner. Hawkins and Shohet (2002) outline the developmental stages of the supervisee as,

Level 1 – self-centred - can I make it in this work?
Level 2 – client centred - can I help this client make it?
Level 3 – process centred – how are we relating together?
Level 4 – process in context centred - how do processes interpenetrate
(p.64)

Supervising beginners

Supervising beginners requires a supervisor to adjust to the beginner's learning needs and be aware of the feelings which a beginner might carry such as: dependence, anxiety, uncertainty, idealisation, initiative, disillusionment, shame, doubt, regression, feel de-skilled and confused and want to be told what to do and how to do it. Research by Stoltenberg and Delworth (1987) identified that the beginner is 'full of trust and hope' (p.49) and motivation, their anxiety is high but they are,

dependent on their supervisor, imitative, neurosis-bound, have an intense self-focus lack self-awareness and other-awareness, often operate from categorical thinking, have some knowledge of theory and skills, but minimal experience' and are seeking the 'right way to do things.

(p.52)

Because beginners are often self-focused they have little internal space to consider and reflect on patient issues. Watkins (2016) considers that beginners need a more structured supervisory environment 'in which they feel properly held and contained and are more actively directed as needed' (p.443) and a supervisory approach that 'is sensitively attuned to their vulnerability' (p.454). In addition, beginners need holding, guidance and validation in their work. Hanoch (2006) advises that new supervisees 'often step into supervision in a heightened state of ambivalence with hopes and expectations as well as fears and anxieties' and that they 'hope to find in the supervisor a person who will appreciate them, show interest and involvement in their work, understand their struggle to learn and grow, and be there for them as a reliable source of guidance and support' (p.132). A beginner may also 'fear … self-exposure to the close observation and criticism of an esteemed other (*the supervisor*). Even constructive and well-intended feedback might feel like criticism and injure the self' (Hanoch, 2006:p.133). All of which indicates the need for the supervisor of beginner therapists to be holding, containing and empathically understanding of the supervisees' anxieties in relation to their new experiences.

Supervising beginners is both rewarding and challenging. Rewarding because as a supervisor you are part of their journey and development as clinicians. Their first experience of supervision will set the groundwork for how they work with patients and consider therapeutic dynamics and unconscious processes. As a result, beginners often require a supervisor to be more active and sometimes directive in enabling them to consider the patient's issues and ways of working analytically and psychodynamically. However, it can be challenging because beginners are often self-focused and confused in relation to theory and practice. Often there is confusion about transference and countertransference. Some beginners think that being a caring mother or father is the transference rather than being open to how the patient perceives them. It can take time for a beginner to realise that transference is about the patient's experience of being parented, which may have been withholding, uncaring or abusive, etc.

Supervising beginners requires providing support, empathy, understanding, input, encouragement, reflection and processing. Sometimes it is helpful for role-play to be used to enable the supervisee to gain a deeper understanding of the patient and the therapeutic processes. In addition, the supervisor needs to model processes of exploration, reflection and an analytic attitude in relation to the patient material and the dynamics of the therapeutic process. Through the supervisory process a beginner will gradually begin to internalise and understand the patient's perspective, inner world, unconscious processes, transference and countertransference and ways of working.

Supervising more experienced supervisees

Supervisees who have some experience will usually have begun to develop their own ideas and developed more internal space to consider self and other but they often still 'vacillate between dependence and autonomy' (Stoltenberg and Delworth, 1987:p.72). To facilitate ongoing supervisee development a supervisor needs to provide a containing and supportive space that enables active exploration and engagement with the patient material and unconscious processes so that the supervisee can reflect on and process their experience. Empathic listening and reflective responses by the supervisor are helpful because they enable the supervisee to feel understood and provide the supervisee with a space to think. It also mirrors an approach to the supervisee as to how to empathically and reflectively listen to the patient and begin to think and imagine the dynamics of the patient's internal world. Reflection and exploration also enable a feedback loop for the supervisee between the supervision and the clinical work because 'whatever the changes that accrue in the therapist during supervision, it is through the therapist's evolving practice self that any such changes are foremost mediated, moderated, maintained, and fortified' (Watkins, 2016: p.444) in relation to the work with the patient.

Experienced supervisees normally have a greater sense of self-awareness and capacity for self-reflection and achieved 'professional identity, mutuality, ability to reflect and more capacity to use their self- and other-awareness' (Stoltenberg and Delworth, 1987:p.95). They also have a greater capacity to think, process and explore unconscious processes and transference and counter-transference in relation to the patient and have an ability to accommodate challenges and to challenge the supervisor (ibid). These latter attributes indicate a more secure ego-related attitude to the work and the capacity to reflect on experience in order to understand the patient.

The learning process

Learning in supervision depends on the supervisory alliance (see Chapter 3), the level of experience of the supervisee and the learning alliance (Flemming and Benedek, 1964, 1966: Watkins, 2015). This requires the supervisor to be 'available, open-minded, honest, reliable, responsive, caring, sensitive, attend to learning needs and supervisee development and provide feedback' (Watkins, 2015: p.462). For a supervisee, learning in supervision can be challenging, frustrating and anxiety provoking but frustration can also be a developmental force. As Bion (1967) states, 'a capacity for tolerating frustration enables the psyche to develop thought as a means by which the frustration that is tolerated is itself made tolerable' (p.112). But this also depends on the supervisee. As del Pozo (1997) comments, learning by the supervisee occurs when they have 'a self with a good-enough capacity to sustain themselves in the fluctuations between "integration-disintegration"'(p.55) because, as del Pozo identifies, learning to be a therapist, or supervisor, can be destabilizing regardless of prior knowledge and experience.

Kernberg (2010), who has written extensively about supervising trainees, considers that 'good supervision is an extremely interesting learning process for both participants' (p.624) and that 'over time, it will become clear to what extent the trainee is developing their own frame of reference' (ibid), integrating theory and practice and developing the clinical skills and competencies of the profession. In a training setting, learning objectives are helpful to clarify what the supervisee and the processes of supervision are working towards. The competencies, identified by Lemma, Roth and Pilling (2008), range from generic therapeutic ones to analytic/dynamic competencies and techniques which include the capacity to process, and work with, transference and countertransference and the dynamics of the therapeutic relationship and develop clinical skills and judgement (p.14).

Working as a supervisor and developing the learning alliance requires evaluating the learning stage of the supervisee (see Chapter 7) so that supervision fits their needs (Watkins, 2015: p.465). It is therefore important for a supervisor to be flexible and attuned to the learning needs of the supervisee rather than expecting the supervisee to fit the attitude and approach of the supervisor or by pathologizing the supervisee for their inability to learn. It is also through exploration of the patient and the session material in supervision that a process becomes modelled by the supervisor and internalised by the supervisee and leads to the generation of their own 'observing ego' (Greenson, 1981) and 'internal supervisor' (Casement, 1985, 1990). This also enables the supervisee to develop their capacity for self-reflection and ability to process and monitor their 'own work from a more detached, *and observing*, internal position' (Stewart, 2002:p.74). The aim of learning in supervision is to enable the development of a competent and self-reflective practitioner who is able to reflect on their experience with the patient, work towards understanding the patient and develop the skills required for therapeutic work.

The professional and the personal

The key component of all psychoanalytic and psychodynamic clinical work is the use of the self in relation to the patient and this is equally true in supervision. Because the learning and development of the supervisee needs to engage the supervisee's internal world psychoanalytic/psychodynamic supervision has been described as 'an activity which is less than personal therapy but more than teaching' (Solnit, 1970:p.360). Frawley O'Dea and Sarnat (2001) comment that

with the contemporary emphasis on the centrality of transference and countertransference in supervision, it is no longer
possible to differentiate the supervisee's professional development from her personal growth, or her professional persona
from her personality. Rather the professional is the personal.

(p.137)

However, they go on to state that 'supervision is most effective
when supervisor and supervisee thoughtfully co-operate in ensuring
that the treat aspect of supervision remains indentured to the over-
arching goal of facilitating the supervisee's growth as a clinician'
(p.140). More recently McWilliams (2021) has commented that,

we do not want to infringe on their analyst's role, but we do
want candidates to understand the myriad ways in which their
personalities, dynamics, histories, and countertransferences
affect their work. The easy answer … is that … supervisory
explorations always return to the patient in treatment. Everything supervisees tell us about their own psychologies should
be bent to the task of helping them with their patients.

(p.142)

This is important because supervision is in the service of the
patient as well as the development of the supervisee. By ensuring
that the focus remains on developing understanding and awareness about the patient the supervisory triangle remains open and
in the service of the professional work and does not collapse into
therapy, even though it may be therapeutic for the supervisee due
to the engagement of their internal world in the process. When
supervision collapses into a two-person relationship without the
presence of the third, the patient, there is a danger of it becoming
therapy rather than supervision.

The professional and personal development of the supervisee
intertwine because real learning in relation to therapeutic work
requires internal, mutative shifts in awareness and perception in
relation to the patient and the experience of being with the
patient. This requires the supervisee to be open to their internal
world so that 'unthought thoughts can be thought about' and 'the

unthinkable' (Driver, 2002:p.58) accessed. This will often challenge and shift the supervisee's own internal objects and patterns of perception. A supervisor therefore 'walks a tightrope between intimacy in relation to the work with the patient and abstinence in terms of the supervisee's own personal work' (Driver, 2002:p.57). This is because the supervisory relationship is formed of the 'psyches of patient, supervisee and supervisor' (Martin, 2002:p.15), but it is the patient who is the focus.

This dynamic came to the fore when a supervisee presented some clinical material in a very agitated, unfocused and distracted way and, as her supervisor, I felt a sense of panic about the supervisee's emotional state. It was important, however, to keep the supervisory triangle open because I did not want it to collapse into a dialogue with the supervisee. I therefore commented that presenting this patient seemed to have stirred up a lot of unsettling feelings about some very difficult events. We were then able to talk and reflect on the impact of the traumatic issues the patient had talked about, which the supervisee had also been affected by. I realised my sense of panic related to both the patient and the supervisee and to the trauma they had experienced, but the focus needed to remain on the patient. In such scenarios the development of the work with the patient and the 'development of the supervisee's professional abilities took place simultaneously' (Driver, 2002:p.54), but they also involved personal shifts for the supervisee. Our discussion about the patient enabled the supervisee to make a connection between the patient material and their own issues, opening up understanding about each, but in the service of the work with the patient.

Resistance and defences against learning in supervision

Resistance and defences against learning in supervision have been written about extensively (Ekstein and Wallerstein, 1958; Kernberg, 1996, 2006, 2007, 2010; Bernard and Goodyear, 1998; Szecsödy, 1989, 1990, 1997; Frawley-O'Dea and Sarnat, 2001; Hawkins and Shohet, 2002; Stewart, 2002; McWilliams, 2021). What is clear is that learning is affected by the supervisee's internal world, attachment styles, defences, anxiety, shame, superego perspectives and the impact of early learning experiences, such as school (Stewart, 2002). These reactions can lead to regression, defences and regression to a more paranoid-schizoid form of functioning. This impedes exploration and influences what is brought to supervision, how it is presented and limits learning, development and understanding about the patient within the supervisee. Narcissistic vulnerabilities, concerns in relation to the supervisor, the clinical material, evaluation by the supervisor, difference (Hanoch, 2006:p.135), and cultural attitudes can also result in defences, disorientation and regression. The supervisor therefore needs to try to understand these phenomena rather than initially blame or pathologize the supervisee. It may emerge that issues need to be addressed in relation to the supervisee's competence, but tackling them directly in the first instance will probably lead to further defences and resistances and risk collapsing supervision into therapy in relation to the supervisee.

Within a training Kernberg (1996, 2006, 2007) points out that a training organisation or a trainer, especially if they are rigid and hierarchical, can generate superego anxieties and defences that inhibit learning because they prevent the supervisee from being open to internal and external exploration with the supervisor. Resistance may relate to the supervisee's anxiety about the training requirements resulting in them focusing on, say, accruing clinical hours rather than the therapeutic alliance and the work with the patient. Kernberg (2006) considers that approaches to training should reflect a more equal partnership between trainee and trainers and that supervision should be a collegial experience as well as one which 'monitors the trainees' work (p.1667). However, Zachrisson (2011) points out the tension in the supervisory relationship between 'the supervisor acting as an authority whilst at the same time trying to foster autonomy in the candidate' (p.947). The attitude of the supervisor is therefore important not only in relation to anxieties generated by training but also those that arise in relation to difference and cultural attitudes (see Chapter 3).

Resistance and defences also lead to some supervisees resorting to what Kadushin (1967/1999) refers to as games in supervision to avoid anxieties. Such games might be the supervisee "seducing" the supervisor by criticising their agency, challenging the supervisor's expertise, deferring to the supervisor, controlling their presentation by coming with a list of issues and redefining the supervisory relationship such as 'protect me or treat me but don't beat me' (p.58). In addition, splitting, seeking approval and avoidance are further ways in which a supervisee may defend against learning and exploration in supervision.

Supervisors can also play games to avoid anxiety and fears. Hawthorne (1975) considers how supervisors can play power and control games by asserting their authority and knowledge and by redefining a supervisee's questioning as resistance. Stimmel (1995) writes about the need for a supervisor to be aware of their own transference dynamics to supervisees and that supervisees can represent a problem or favourite because they link to the supervisor's own history and internal world. In addition, Stimmel also points out the danger of a supervisor falling into the trap of 'narcissistic gratification when their comments result in positive feedback and intellectually pleasing results' (Driver, 2023:p.8).

Learning can also be inhibited by dumb spots, blind spots and deaf spots (Ekstein and Wallerstein, 1958; Szecsödy, 1989). Dumb spots refer to the lack of 'knowledge, information and skill (not due to resistance)' whereas blind spots are 'due to a defensive avoidance of information' (Szecsödy, 1989:p.250). Deaf spots refer to when the supervisee/therapist is unable to hear the patient or supervisor due to their own defences and resistance. All will influence how the supervisee learns and relates to the supervisor and supervision.

Learning and the superego

Processes of learning and exploration in supervision also rely on the supervisor and supervisee relating in an adult-to-adult, ego-to-ego way, but this is often not the case, especially when the superego comes into play. Beginners to clinical work are often focused on the right way to do things and even more experienced supervisees might experience anxiety about being competent, not getting things right or 'not being as good as they had hoped' (Driver, 2019:p.160). The superego can therefore become a powerful inhibitor of learning because it can act as a censor and persecutor (Driver, 2023) especially when issues of the patient touch on areas the supervisee is uncomfortable with or defends against (see Chapter 4).

Superego dynamics became apparent in the work of one supervisee when he constantly interspersed his presentations with comments such as "I shouldn't have said that" and "I know you will say I did it wrong". As a result, it became very difficult to explore with him what had actually been presented by the patient, his responses or his countertransference feelings. I commented that I felt he was being very hard on himself and wondered what it felt like for him working with this patient. I hoped that my empathic and benign response might enable him to open up about the work. Gradually he was able to comment that he criticised himself so as to avoid others (me) criticising him, but he also realised that this prevented exploration. His responses indicated that his persecutory superego linked to both his personal and professional self but in supervision our exploration remained focused on his professional self and the work with his patients. Slowly this shifted something in him and we were able to work towards a more benign and open way of considering and processing the dynamics that evolved in his clinical work.

When a supervisor can enable and foster a benign superego and an ego-related position with the supervisee, states of unknowing can be sustained, mistakes considered, open and flexible exploration generated and true internal learning can occur.

Learning in individual supervision and group supervision

The dynamics of learning in supervision also depends on whether supervision is individual or in a group. Individual supervision holds the potential for a more detailed and focused exploration, which allows the supervisor and the supervisee to consider the clinical material in detail intra-psychically as well as inter-personally and explore feelings, transference, countertransference, hypothesise about the patient's internal world and consider issues of technique. However, in individual supervision, the interaction is more direct, which may activate defences and retreats from the more intense exposure that one-to-one supervision can bring.

In a group setting the group dynamics will affect the supervisee and their attitude to learning (see Chapter 3). However, the learning cycle of observation, reflection and thought (Kolb, 1984: Kolb and

Kolb, 2005) can make good use of the group dynamics and the experiences of all supervisees because each supervisee is affected, consciously and unconsciously, by the patient material presented. For example, the presentation of a depressed, passive patient may elicit an angry response in one of the members of the group. Exploration of this affect, and hypotheses about what it might link to for the patient, can usefully open up awareness and understanding.

To enable learning in either individual or group supervision the supervisor needs to be aware of the dynamics of each and to work appropriately and sensitively in either. What is important to hold in mind is that supervision is about a third, the patient, and that the learning processes of supervision revolves around developing the supervisees' understanding of the patient and the development of their clinical skills.

Supervision and ongoing learning

Learning in supervision is not just about developing competencies, it is also about learning the skills to be an effective practitioner and realising that learning is an ongoing process throughout the professional career of the practitioner. The requirements of continuing professional development (CPD) and supervision following qualification (requirements in many countries) is a recognition that blind spots in relation to unconscious processes are inevitable and that learning in relation to clinical skills and the patient is continuous. Such a perspective also recognises that learning as a clinician is not just about learning to decode and understand the patient material it is also about developing ways to work effectively with patients. Yakely (2014) cites research that demonstrates the efficacy of psychoanalytic and psychodynamic therapies and although as therapists and supervisors we may not work directly with outcome measures we all have a sense of whether a therapy is working effectively for the patient. It is therefore important for a supervisor to reflectively consider issues of technique and clinical skills with their supervisees.

Within supervision it is also vital to ensure that a clinician does not stagnate or passively go through the motions in terms of learning and practice. Rousmaniere et al. (2017) outlines the importance of what they term deliberate practice in which super-vision provides 'feedback, addresses knowledge and skills deficits and challenges' (p.9). Their concept of deliberate practice recognises that it is all too easy for a qualified clinician to slip into comfortable ways of thinking and working and that both supervisor and supervisee need to take deliberate steps to confront and develop learning in relation to the patient and the skills of being a clinician. Deliberate practice relates to the attitude of both supervisor and supervisee and identifies how a supervisor and supervision provide ongoing developmental and learning processes.

Final reflection on supervision and learning

Learning in supervision aims to enable the supervisee to process their experience with their patient and learn how to interweave theory and practice, develop a reflective ego that is open to exploration, develop the capacity to step into the unknown (think the unthinkable) and reflect on, and make use, of unconscious processes in the work with the patient. 'When supervision goes well, it is alive, vibrant and vibrating with the cognitive, linguistic, affective, somatic, and relational responses of supervisee and supervisor to the patient and to one another' (Frawley O'Dea and Sarnat, 2001:p.70). It is within, and through, the supervisory relationship that the supervisee develops as a clinician and learning occurs. But a supervisee needs to combine theory and experience, and Bolognini (2019) raises the important point that it is not the therapist's theoretical orientation that is important 'but rather what "happens in most therapists" minds when they engage, on the one hand with a clinical situation, and on the other with the theoretical assumptions to which they adhere' (p.11). This is because 'each individual therapist builds, inhabits, and utilises a unique internal laboratory when he or she interacts with patients' (ibid) – a dynamic equally important between supervisor and supervisee.

In order to achieve such a synthesis of theory and practice, a supervisor may need to be, from time to time, facilitator, 'teacher, mentor, reliable other' (Collens and van Hout, 2017) as well as occupy the role of 'monitoring, safeguarding and evaluating competence' (Stewart, 2002) in relation to the standards and skills of the profession. A key aim of supervision is to enable learning in the supervisee about the patient and the development of their professional skills. Sensitivity and awareness to the learning stage and learning needs of the supervisee is, therefore, a key factor in the work of the supervisor.

References

Bernard, J.M. and Goodyear, R.K. (1998) *Fundamentals of Clinical Supervision. Second Edition*. London and Toronto: Allyn and Bacon.

Bion, W.R. (1967) *Second Thoughts*. New York: Aronson.

Bolognini, S. (2019) 'Enchantments and disenchantments in the formation and use of psychoanalytic theories about psychic reality'. *Ital. Psychoanal. Annu.* (13):11–24.

Casement, P. (1985) *On Learning from the Patient*. London: Tavistock Publications.

Casement, P. (1990) *Further Learning From the Patient*. London: Routledge.

Collens, P. and van Hout, F. (2017) 'Learning in psychotherapy group supervision: Transcending complementarity and the generative potential of group conflict'. *Brit. J. Psychother.* (33)(2):177–191.

del Pozo, M.M. (1997) 'On the process of supervision in psychoanalytic Psychotherapy'. Martindale, B., *et al.* (eds.) *Supervision and Its Vicissitudes*. London: Karnac Books.

Driver, C. (2002) 'Internal states in the supervisory relationship'. Driver, C. and Martin, E. (eds.) *Supervising Psychotherapy: Psychoanalytic and Psychodynamic Perspectives*. London: Sage.

Driver, C. (2019) 'The superego as a significant factor in clinical training'. Harding, C. (ed.) *Dissecting the Superego*. London: Routledge.

Driver, C. (2023) 'The superego in supervision. Censor, persecutor or protector'. *Psychodynamic Practice*. https://doi.org/10.1080/14753634.2023.2282721.

Ekstein, R. and Wallerstein, R.S. (1958) *The Teaching and Learning of Psychotherapy*. Madison Connecticut: International Universities Press, Inc.

Fleming, J. and Benedek, T. F. (1964) 'Supervision. A method of teaching psychoanalysis'. *The Psychoanalytic Quarterly* (33):71–96.

Fleming, J. and Benedek, T. F. (1966) *Psychoanalytic Supervision*. New York, NY: Grune & Stratton.

Frawley-O'Dea, M.G. and Sarnat, J.E. (2001) *The Supervisory Relationship*. New York: The Guilford Press.

Greenson, R.R. (1981) *The Technique and Practice of Psychoanalysis.* London: Hogarth Press.

Hanoch, E. (2006) 'The loudness of the unspoken: Candidates' anxiety in supervision'. *Psychoanal. Persp.* (3)(2):127–146.

Hawkins, P. and Shohet, R. (2002) *Supervision in the Helping Professions,* 2nd edition. Buckingham and Philadelphia: Open University Press.

Hawthorne, L. (1975) 'Games supervisors play'. *Social Work* (20)(3), May 1975:179–183. https://doi.org/10.1093/sw/20.3.179.

Jung, C.G. (1921) *Psychological Types CW6.* London: Routledge. 1989.

Kadushin, A. (1967/1999) 'Games People Play in Supervision'. *Reflections: Narratives of Professional Helping* (5)(3):55–64. https://reflectionsnarrativesofprofessionalhelping.org/index.php/Reflections/article/view/624 (Accessed 05. 01. 2021).

Kernberg, O.F. (1996) 'Thirty methods to destroy the creativity of psychoanalytic candidates'. *International Journal of Psychoanalysis* (77):1031–1040.

Kernberg, O.F. (2006) 'The coming changes in psychoanalytic education: Part 1'. *International Journal of Psychoanalysis* (87):1649–1673.

Kernberg, O.F. (2007) 'The coming changes in psychoanalytic education: Part 11'. *International Journal of Psychoanalysis* (88):183–202.

Kernberg, O.F. (2010) 'Psychoanalytic supervision: The supervisor's tasks'. *Psychoanal. Q.,* (79)(3):603–627.

Kolb, D.A. (1984) *Learning Styles.* http://changingminds.org/explanations/learning/kolb_learning.htm (Accessed 6. 1. 2024).

Kolb, D.A. (2015) *Experiential Learning. Experience as the Source of Learning and Development.* 2nd edition. New Jersey: Pearson Education, Inc.

Kolb, A.Y. and Kolb, D.A. (2005) 'The Kolb learning style inventory—Version 3.1 technical specifications'. https://www.researchgate.net/publication/241157771 29.1.2024 (Accessed 6. 1. 2024).

Lemma, A., Roth, A.D. and Pilling, S. (2008) 'The competences required to deliver effective Psychoanalytic/Psychodynamic Therapy. Research Department of Clinical, Education and Health Psychology. University College London (UCL)'. https://www.researchgate.net/publication/237553451_The_Competences_Required_to_Deliver_Effective_PsychoanalyticPsychodynamic_Therapy (Accessed 6. 1. 2024).

Martin, E. (2002) 'Listening to the absent patient'. Driver, C. and Martin, E. (eds.) *Supervising Psychotherapy.* London: Sage Publications.

McWilliams, N. (2021) *Psychoanalytic Supervision.* New York and London: The Guilford Press.

Myers, J.B. (1962) *The Myers-Briggs Type Indicator.* Palo Alto, CA: Consulting Psychologists Press.

Piaget, J. (1958) *The Development of Thought: Equilibration of Cognitive Structures.* New York: Viking.

Rousmaniere, T., Goodyear, R. K., Miller, S. D. and Wampold, B. E. (eds) (2017) *The Cycle of Excellence: Using Deliberate Practice to Improve Supervision and Training.* New Jersey and West Sussex: Wiley-Blackwell.

Solnit, A. (1970) 'Learning from psychoanalytic supervision'. *Inter. J. Psychoanal,* (51)(3):359–362.

Stewart, J. (2002) 'The interface between teaching and supervision'. Driver, C. and Martin, E. (eds), *Supervising Psychotherapy.* London: Sage Publications.

Stimmel, B. (1995) 'Resistance to awareness of the supervisor's transference with special reference to the parallel process'. *Int. J. Psychoanal.* 76(6):609–618.

Stoltenberg, C.D. and Delworth, U. (1987) *Supervising Counselors and Therapists.* San Francisco and London: Jossey-Bass.

Szecsödy, I. (1989) 'Supervision: A didactic or mutative situation'. *Psychoanal. Psychother.* (4)(3): 245–261.

Szecsödy, I. (1990) *The Learning Process in Psychotherapy Supervision.* Stockholm: Department of Psychiatry, Karolinska Institutet, St Gorans Hospital.

Szecsödy, I. (1997) '(How) is learning possible in supervision?' Martindale, B.*et al.* (eds.) *Supervision and its Vicissitudes.* London: Karnac Books.

Szecsödy, I. (2013) 'Supervision should be a mutual learning experience'. *Scand. Psychoanal. Rev.* (36)(2):126–129.

Thomas, S. (2005) 'Supervision and training: two different foci'. Driver, C. and Martin, E. (eds.) *Supervision and the Analytic Attitude.* London: Whurr.

Watkins, C.E. (2013) 'On psychoanalytic supervisor competencies, the persistent paradox without parallel in psychoanalytic education, and dreaming of an evidence-based psychoanalytic supervision'. *Psychoanal. Rev.* (100)(4):609–646.

Watkins, C.E. (2015) 'The learning alliance in psychoanalytic supervision. A fifty-year retrospective and prospective'. *Psychoanal. Psychol.* (32)(3):451–481.

Watkins, C.E. (2016) 'Listening, learning, and development in psychoanalytic supervision: A self psychology perspective'. *Psychoanal. Psychol.* (33)(3):437–471.

Watkins, C.E. and Scaturo, D. (2014) 'Proposal for a common language, educationally informed model of psychoanalytic supervision'. *Psychoanal. Inq.* (34)(6):619–633.

Yakeley, J. (2014) 'Psychodynamic psychotherapy: Developing the evidence base'. *Advances in Psychiatric Treatment* (20):269–279. doi:10.1192/apt.bp.113.012054.

Zachrisson, A. (2011) 'Dynamics of psychoanalytic supervision: A heuristic model'. *Int. J. Psychoanal.* (92)(4):943–961.

Chapter 6

Listening, exploring and interpreting in supervision

When a supervisee presents their clinical work in supervision there are a number of different dimensions to listen to, reflect on and explore. Hawkins and Shohet (2002) itemise seven points that a supervisor needs to engage with:

- 'the content of the therapy session;
- the strategies and interventions used by the therapist;
- the therapy process and relationship;
- the therapist's countertransference;
- the here-and-now process as a mirror or parallel of the there-and-then process;
- the supervisor's countertransference;
- the wider context of the work'.(pp.69–71)

All of these perspectives need consideration and what a supervisor hears can be influenced by any one of them. This raises the question of how we listen to our supervisee's presentation and how we respond in words that generate reflective thought and understanding in the supervisee.

Listening

What we hear as a supervisor depends on our attitude and orientation. If we maintain free floating attention when we listen to, and observe, the presentation of a supervisee, we are more open to hearing, and picking up, the non-verbal and unconscious

DOI: 10.4324/9781003496137-6

communications as well as the verbal, conscious ones. Ogden (1999) identifies that listening needs to involve being receptive to primary process unconscious communication and not just conscious (secondary process) communication. In addition, listening in supervision requires pre-reflective, non-linear thinking (Yerushalmi, 2024a:p.25) and free-floating associative dream thought along with directed, reality-based, thinking (Jung, 1911–12/1952: para.17) so as to connect both conscious and unconscious communications. Listening in supervision is, therefore, a multi-layered activity (Ogden, 2005) and, based on Ogden's work, Zachrisson (2011) comments that this involves 'listening to the session report, the transference and resistance in the session, the countertransference, noticed and unnoticed, by the supervisee and the process in the supervisory situation itself, including the countertransference reactions of the supervisor' (Zachrisson, 2011:p.953).

A supervisor therefore needs to listen to the conscious content of the supervisee's presentation and the patient's material and, in a state of reverie (Bion, 1967), be open to the unconscious communications and the unthinkable, the O (Bion, 1970), that arise during the process of supervision in relation to the presented patient. Ogden (1999), reflecting on Bion's (ibid) work comments that reverie is, 'our ruminations, daydreams, fantasies, bodily sensations, fleeting perceptions, images emerging from states of half-sleep, tunes, and phrases that run through our minds, and so on' (p.158). Reverie in supervision can generate an image, a symbol, that represents something important about the work and the patient. This can enable the creation of hypotheses about the patient and the dynamics of the session in the safe and boundaried space of supervision. Yorke (2005) comments that 'typical of the experience of reverie is that while the supervisee is making their presentation the supervisor may become engrossed in a preoccupying interlude which has captured his or her mind' (p.39). As a result a selected fact may emerge which throws light on the internal world of the patient, their patterns of relating and the transference dynamics with their therapist/supervisee. However, Britton and Steiner (1994) highlight that when listening to patients (or supervisees) it is important to ensure we don't get seduced by an 'overvalued idea' but find an observation that links and integrates disparate facts into a 'meaningful pattern', leading to 'the emergence of a selected fact' (p.1070). Yorke (2005) reflects that 'the accurate identification of the selected fact cannot be overemphasised. The temptation to self-indulgence in the reveries is one of the risks inherent in the method' (p.49).

Reverie, and its links to imagination, are an important part of how we listen in supervision and Bravesmith (2008) comments that 'the contents of the undifferentiated matrix (*of supervision*) emerges through imaginative activity, before being subjected to rational secondary process, thinking' (p.106). However, imagination can be limited if the focus of the process is on defining and Gee (1996) comments that the supervisory process needs to be 'relating, then defining' (p.529) and Ogden (1999) 'draws attention to the stifling effect on imagination of our efforts to define' (p.3). This is because imagination and understanding needs to engage the supervisee's mind so that thoughts, ideas and images come alive, or become irrelevant, when they are explored in relation to the patient.

Exploring

The challenge of supervision is that listening and exploration is in relation to an absent patient who is presented in supervision through the medium of the supervisee (Martin, 2002). Ogden (2005) writes about the importance of the supervisor facilitating the supervisee in 'dreaming up' the patient (p.1267) in supervision and considers that the patient 'presented is a fiction created in the medium of words, voice, physical movement (e.g., the supervisee's hand gestures), irony, wit, unconscious communications such as projective identification, and so on' (p.1267). The patient presented is, therefore, a representation conveyed by the supervisee. Exploration and brainstorming with the supervisee enables the examination of different hypotheses about the patient, their inner world and the transference and countertransference dynamics within the therapy. Gee comments on the importance of pondering between supervisor and supervisee so that 'dialogue takes place between the conscious and unconscious parts of the self' (Gee, 1996:p.540) and engages the mind and inner world of the supervisee and supervisor in relation to the patient. Pondering also links to the importance of uncertainty. Interpretations in supervision are not about presenting a certainty but about generating inner thought in the listener because 'if the supervisor defines too much then the supervisee is prevented from relating to, and interacting with, their experience' (Driver, 2005:p.29). Winnicott (1980) was of the view that interpretations need to convey the limits of understanding (p.102) so as to create the chance to play with ideas and Bollas comments that interpretations, 'are appreciated less for their content, and more for their function as structuring experiences' (Bollas, 1991:p.21). Such approaches enable the supervisee to find their own perspective and understanding.

The nature of exploration in supervision also links to how we orientate our thinking. Jacobs et al. (1995) identifies four types of thinking 'inductive, associative, creative and self-reflective' (p.59) as particularly important in supervision because they are dynamically oriented. Crawford (2005) focuses specifically on free association and associative thought and, adapting Bollas's (2002:p.37) ideas, writes that 'the method of free association subverts the supervisor's natural authoritarian tendencies' (Crawford, 2005: p.58) because 'free association is an expansive process' (p.56) and the 'product of two minds at work' (Kris, 1996:p.ix). Crawford (2005) goes on to comment that in an

> associative way of working, whether it be one-to-one or in a group, a situation is created in which insights can arise as part of a process, and not necessarily from the person who is the most experienced, in a way that can feel collaborative, perhaps involving a form of play.
>
> (p. 58)

Crawford concludes that free association facilitates 'the development of the supervisee and also of the supervisor and, through their joint efforts, helps develop the therapeutic work with, and for the benefit of, the patient' (Crawford, 2005:p.59).

Exploration also involves intuition, curiosity and the capacity to play with ideas in relation to the patient and the therapeutic relationship. Kernberg (2010) comments that intuition 'is a form of rapid processing of unconscious and preconscious components from within the theoretical frame of reference in which the supervisor has been trained' (p.605). He proposes combining and integrating issues of theory and technique with intuitive responses so as to 'capture the communication of unconscious meaning from patient to supervisee, from supervisee to supervisor, and from the supervisor to both supervisee and patient in terms of his or her countertransference reaction' (ibid:p.605). Encouraging intuition, curiosity and play within the supervisee, also enables a connection between dream thinking and directed thinking and facilitates supervisees to find their own connections and thoughts about the patient material. Kernberg (2010) writes that the supervisor's explorations and self-reflection models a process for the supervisee and facilitates the development of the supervisee's own 'self-reflective attitude' (p.625). Such explorations may lead to uncertainty and frustration, but result in the supervisee's capacity to think, process and make sense of the conscious and unconscious communications and sensory experiences in the work with the patient.

Exploring in supervision is essential but it can be hampered if the supervisor is too closely attached to theory. Böhm (2002) reflects on the difference between 'analytic appliers versus analytic explorers' (p.20) in which the latter 'is an explorer of unknown territory' in which 'there is always something more to explore, something we do not understand' (p.20). He goes on to comment that exploration can be obstructed by the temptation to order and categorise the clinical material prematurely in relation to theory especially if we remain focused on our own theoretical constructs rather than be open to new experiences and discoveries and the supervisee's association and ideas. However, exploration in supervision is not always a straightforward process. Defences in either supervisee or supervisor can impede thinking (see Chapters 4 and 5) especially when patient issues, conscious and unconscious, link to problems and defences within the supervisee or supervisor. It is therefore important to be aware of issues that are avoided and not spoken about so as to bring into thought the unthinkable or the unbearable. Sometimes therefore the role of the supervisor is to think the unthinkable and to use this to develop both insight and understanding with, and for, the supervisee in relation to the patient.

Exploration, curiosity, free association and pondering, when used in an open and reflective way between supervisor and supervisee, are ways in which the supervisory space can be used creatively to generate understanding and awareness about the patient and their internal world. But such exploratory processes require words and language so it is important to consider how we put our ideas and thoughts into words.

Language, communication and responding in supervision

Supervision is a 'space for thought' (Nagell et al., 2014:p.574) and reflection and, based on Winnicott's ideas (1979, 1980), an intermediate space in which thoughts and ideas can be created between the supervisor and supervisee. But we explore and relate with our supervisees primarily through our words so it is important to consider how the words we use motivate the supervisee into their own reflections and thoughts. 'Words name, act or describe; they link, connect and create movement; they give both cognitive and emotional impact' (Driver, 2005: p.20) and have the potential to touch the internal world of the listener, the supervisee, and take them on a journey that engages external and internal dialogues. Ogden, citing William James' ideas, comments that 'language fails to convey meaning (especially affective meaning) when it is used in a fashion that is focused on what it is saying as opposed to what it is doing' (Ogden 1999:225). That is, we need to consider not only what our words say, but also what they do to the listener, the supervisee, and whether they create understanding, perceptual shifts and awareness. Vygotsky (2002) comments that, 'words and other signs are those means that direct our mental operations, control their course, and channel them toward the solution of the problem confronting us' (p.106). However, he goes on to point out that, 'thought is not begotten by thought; it is engendered by motivation, i.e., by our desires and needs, our interests and our emotions' (p.254).

It is therefore vital to consider what our words do to the listener and whether they motivate the supervisee into their own thinking and exploration. That is, do our words just impart information or do they take the supervisee 'on a journey that engages external and internal dialogues' and 'create those aha moments that shift understanding and assumptions' (Driver, 2005:p.20)? As a supervisor it is therefore important to be aware that there are different ways in which we can interact and engage with our supervisees. These can range from didactic interactions to reflections and explorations of the patient material. Being mindful of how we interact with our supervisees helps us be aware of the dynamics we create and work with. The different styles of supervisory interaction and our use of language, all of which are needed from time to time, include,

a   Didactic or directive communication; a one-person mode of interaction in which the supervisor gives the supervisee information or ideas about theory or the patient. Such communication is focused on the supervisor's perspective rather than a dialogue with the supervisee about their thoughts and ideas. Didactic or directive communication limits the involvement of the supervisee and their thinking and processing but it is important if theory or issues around clinical technique, clinical responsibility, assessment of a trainee's progress or fitness to practice issues need to be addressed.

b   Dialogue; a two-person dynamic in which the thoughts, ideas and understandings of both supervisor and supervisee are explored in order to reconstruct and understand the patient's inner world and patterns of relating. When there is a mutual recognition of each other's views (Yerushalmi, 2024b) dialogue enables the supervisee to develop their own ideas and sense of professional identity. However, dialogue can lead to discussion about the patient rather than exploration of the impact of the patient material on the therapist/supervisee and the supervisor in terms of transference, countertransference and parallel process.

c   Interactive and reflective communication; based on the three-person dynamic of patient, therapist/supervisee and supervisor it includes conceptualisations and reflections on any parallel process phenomena within supervision in relation to the patient material. This involves the supervisor gathering up, and internally reflecting on, the patient material, the supervisee's presentation, the style of interaction with the supervisee and transference and countertransference phenomena between patient and therapist and between the supervisee and themselves. Reflection on this by the supervisor to the supervisee, in relation to the patient material, can enable the engagement of the supervisee's inner world and develop awareness and a deeper understanding about the patient.

For example, a supervisee, Omar, presented a patient whom he described as depressed following the recent death of his wife. As Omar spoke about the session I felt an intense sense of sadness, but frustration at Omar's matter-of-fact way of speaking about the patient and his focus on wanting the patient to move on. I was surprised at the lack of emotion in the presentation and felt concern about the apparent disconnect between the patient material and the manner in which it was conveyed by Omar. As I reflected on this I wondered if there were links or any parallel process in relation to the patient. I commented to Omar that I felt that the patient was bringing a lot of difficult and painful material about his wife's death and his experience of her dying but wondered if it was hard to listen to. Omar said he was irritated by the way the patient kept going over and over the details of his wife's death, but never showed any emotion when talking about it. I said the patient's lack of emotion and Omar's feelings of annoyance were interesting and that it felt as if the patient was avoiding getting in touch with his feelings. Omar was thoughtful and started to talk about how the patient had been very dependent on his wife and that perhaps he felt helpless now that she had died but was ashamed to admit it. I went on to ask Omar what he felt when he was with the patient. Omar said he found it hard to admit how annoyed and frustrated he felt. I commented that perhaps the patient was angry with his wife for dying. This enabled Omar to consider a wider range of issues in relation to the patient and the difficulty for the patient to get in touch with his feelings and mourn the loss of his wife.

The importance of these explorations with Omar, based on a triangular dynamic and parallel process, were that it enabled a reflective space to develop in which we could both explore. This was also facilitated by Omar's experience as a psychotherapist. Working with parallel process requires the supervisee to have attained a self-reflective capacity whereas a 'supervisee new to clinical work may not have the capacity to internalise, twin-track and reflect on the simultaneous input of the patient material and the supervisor's interpretations' (Driver, 2005:p.25) and may need more directive exploration. However, when the supervisor does reflect on parallel process and the triangular dynamic of supervision, it mirrors a process to the supervisee about how unconscious processes and issues from the patient can be reflected on and generates a deeper understanding of the patient and their internal world.

d   Reflecting from a meta-perspective; reflecting and interpreting in relation to the impact on the supervisory and clinical work of all aspects of the clinical rhombus including the context such as private practice, in an organisation, in person or online. This is especially relevant when organisational or external factors impact on the clinical and supervisory work. For example, when an organisation makes changes, such as its fee, this has both conscious and unconscious implications for all and will emerge as a motif, explicitly or implicitly, in the patient material or the supervisee's presentation. External events such as war, violence, political unrest or the Covid pandemic also impact on both clinical and supervisory work. Such events can generate anxiety and this can ripple through the whole system of patient, therapist/supervisee and supervisor.

Reflecting on the dynamics of the clinical rhombus is important and requires a supervisor to develop an attitude of mind that can rotate through, and reflect on, the impact of the dynamics emanating from the patient, the therapist/supervisee, the supervisor and the context. Juggling these perspectives can enable a fifth, or meta-perspective, to emerge (Figure 6.1) (Driver, 2020:p.131). Being able to reflect and interpret from this perspective enables a more holistic view to be considered in relation to the patient and the dynamics of the clinical work. Awareness of this in terms of the clinical rhombus and considering such issues and dynamics from a meta-perspective

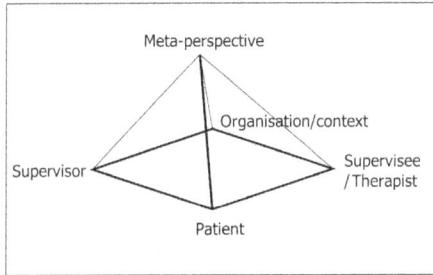

Figure 6.1 A Meta-perspective
Source: Driver (2020)

provides both supervisor and supervisee with the capacity to separate out the underlying issues and generate a greater depth of understanding in relation to the work with the patient.

Our style of communication with our supervisees is important and we need to be aware of how we are interacting with them but sometimes it is also important to consider when 'to stay quietly by and allow the satisfaction the worker (*therapist*) is obtaining in a twosome with the client' (Mattinson, 1997:p.12). In our interactions with our supervisees it is therefore important to find forms of intervention that facilitate the development of the self-reflecting capacity of the supervisee, mentalization and the internalisation of a supervisory attitude.

The aim of listening, exploring and interpreting in supervision

As supervisors, we also need to consider the aims of our interventions and what we are hoping to achieve. In supervision we are aiming to generate a deeper understanding in the supervisee about the patient and also enable the supervisee's development as a clinician and their capacity for reflective processing. Our use of words can generate insight, awareness, internal shifts in understanding and create meaning. Steele (1979) comments that understanding 'arises in dialectical and linguistic interactions with other people and the world; ... past experiences, current intentions, and future expectations all shape understanding' (p.391). Steele, commenting on the hermeneutic[1] cycle, goes on to state that 'understanding involves a continuous circular movement from the parts to the whole and back again from the whole to its parts' (p.392) in which 'the goal of interpretation is to arrive at a meaning which maximises the understanding of the parts in terms of the whole' (p.392). This enables the creation of shared meaning in relation to the patient. Understanding and finding meaning is therefore achieved through dialogue, internally and relationally, and rests on the context of each specific encounter. It requires the interplay of subjectivity and objectivity and an openness to diversity, difference and the reality of each encounter. The implications of this is that we should never make assumptions about a patient or supervisee but listen and interpret in relation to the material presented and the experience of each supervisee's presentation.

A supervisor's exploration and dialogue with a supervisee also facilitates the development of inner speech (Vygotsky, 2002) and inner dialogue about the patient within the supervisee. This enables the development of a professional self and an internal supervisor (Casement, 1985, 1990). Our interventions as a supervisor therefore need to engage the ego of the supervisee so as to enable them to develop their own observing ego (Greenson, 1981), which can reflect on, and explore, their experience of, and with, the patient and the patient's patterns of relating. Such processes require experiential learning, learning from experience (Casement, 1985) and mentalization. Fonagy et al., (2012) describe mentalization as, 'the imaginative mental activity that enables us to perceive and interpret human behaviour in terms of internal mental states (e.g., needs, desires, feelings, beliefs, goals, purposes and reasons etc.,)' (p.4). It 'involves perceiving and interpreting the feelings, thoughts, beliefs, and wishes that explain what people do ... and ... entails an awareness of someone else's circumstances, his or her prior patterns of behaviour, and the experiences to which the individual has been exposed' (Fonagy and Bateman, 2019:p.3) – a perspective vital to supervisee and supervisor alike.

Our words, and the way they are received by the supervisee are important. A supervisee who is a passive listener may rely on the supervisor to do the work and not engage internally with the patient material resulting only, at best, cognitive understanding. But, if our words and explorations engage the supervisee's mind they can motivate them into their own thinking, reflecting and reverie about the patient and enable emotional and internal learning and understanding.

Moments of meeting

Engaging the mind of the supervisee in exploration about the patient and the session material enables their insight and awareness to develop. Based on the work of Stern et al., (1998) and the Boston Change Process Study Group (2013) Yerushalmi (2018) considers the importance of moments of meeting in supervision. These moments of meeting may be verbal or non-verbal such as 'a belly laugh, an empathic look, a shared moment of sadness, or an unexpected non-verbal exchange' (Gabbard, 2000:p.14) and are 'unplanned, spontaneous, transformational and expand the participants' consciousness' (Stern et al., 1998:p.904). Yerushalmi points out that such moments of meeting in supervision shifts the role of the supervisor from being a commentator on the work with the patient to a dynamic in which both supervisor and supervisee 'co-construct meanings and plan therapeutic actions together' (p.237). To achieve this requires the supervisor to allow, from time to time, a more relaxed atmosphere in supervision so as to 'loosen up the boundaries between themselves and their supervisees and allow the interpenetration of both partners' minds and facilitate their perception that "I know that you know that I know," which characterizes moments of meeting' (Stern, 2004:p.75 in Yerushalmi, 2018:p.239).

Yerushalmi (2018) also considers the challenge and limitations of such interactions in terms of boundaries and the possible assessment role of the supervisor in relation to supervisees. But he goes on to comment that although 'the supervisory framework, with its ground rules and specific roles assigned to each participant, is vital for supervision' (p.242) stepping out of the assigned roles from time to time, can create a highly important propelling force to expand and deepen the supervisory work. Supervisors' consent to step out of their formal roles temporarily, only to return to them later and establish them further, frees their supervisees' minds, as well as their own, to think more creatively. The more the supervisory framework is internalized and becomes symbolically represented in the supervisors' minds, the easier it is for them to break it temporarily and then reestablish it and resume their assigned roles.

(Yerushalmi, 2018:p.242)

Being aware of how we relate to our supervisees therefore helps us consider the involvement of the supervisee in the process of understanding the patient and the dynamics of the work. Our words, our style of interventions and our moments of meeting can facilitate this.

Neuroscience and language

Neuroscience has provided insight into therapeutic and supervisory interactions. However, research into the brain/mind, and its application within the therapeutic field, is a vast area of study and I will only briefly touch on some of the findings here.

Pally (2003) identifies that 'during verbal interactions with others, the brain generates symbolic categories such as self, non-self, actions, images, even its own internal sensations, and relates them to ongoing events of primary consciousness' (p.167). A perspective that reinforces psychoanalytic theories about the dynamic interaction between the unconscious and the conscious. Gabbard (2000) warns, however, that the 'language of the mind and the language of the brain are quite different' and 'that mind and brain, while never separate from one another, cannot be fully integrated either' (p.3). But he goes on to comment on their interconnectivity and that 'emotion, perception, thought, memory, and behaviour are all the product of activated neural circuits' (ibid:p.4). Neural circuits being a circuit of interconnecting neurons (nerve cells) that send messages through the brain and the body.

Westen and Gabbard (2002a, 2002b) examine neuroscience in relation to memory and highlight that cognitive processing is not linear because 'at every moment, we are inundated with sensory information, not to mention our own thoughts and feelings' (Westen and Gabbard, 2002a:p.65). In addition they describe how when we listen and hear a sentence, 'information processing occurs in parallel, outside of awareness' (p.73) and that this is subject to activation or inhibition in which 'every act of thought and memory is simultaneously an act of affect regulation' (p.92). These findings resonate with many psychoanalytic theories and thinking. They also highlight the interrelationship between the psychological and the physiological and the impact of language in the therapeutic or supervisory relationship. In a later paper, Gabbard and Westen (2003) consider the difference between cognitive, conscious processing and unconscious, implicit ones. They comment that cognitive neuroscience suggests, 'implicit processes are psychologically and neurologically distinct from explicit ones, so that targeting only those processes that reach conscious awareness is likely to leave many important associational networks untouched' (p.830). This has implications for our use of language with our supervisees and reinforces the importance of being aware of how our words affect them.

Schore's (2012) research explores this further. He considers that 'the left and right hemispheres … of the brain … process information in their own unique fashion' (p.119). The left brain being primarily a conscious system with a language and cognitive focus and the right brain an unconscious and emotional processing system responding to non-verbal, emotional and empathic communication. The right brain also contains implicit memory, responds to implicit communication and 'moment-to-moment right brain-to-right brain' (p.129) visual, auditory, emotionally charged and unconscious communications with others. Schore's ideas have implications for our responses as analysts, therapists and supervisors and links to Piaget's (1958) and Szecsödy's (1990, 1997) identification of the difference between cognitive and emotional understanding. If there is an implicit and unconscious resistance in communication between the left brain and right brain cognitive understanding will not create insight or emotional and perceptual shifts. Whereas emotional and empathic communication, which impacts on the right brain, enables deeper levels of insight, awareness and understanding. This brings us back to the need to be aware of what our words do to our supervisees. Do our words just link to cognitive understanding or do they lead the supervisee to insight and perceptual shifts that might even result in 'restructuring the unconscious itself' (Schore, 2012:p.143)?

Things unsaid in supervision

What we consciously hear, focus on or speak about is influenced by defences, repression and unconscious processes. It is therefore important to reflect on what is not spoken about or mentioned in supervision. This might be something obvious such as focusing on issues relating to the father of the patient and not speaking about the mother. Awareness of this will immediately identify what is absent from the narrative about the patient and enable exploration of this missing dimension. However, often what is not spoken about in supervision remains hidden because it links to shame or defences in the patient, supervisee and possibly the supervisor. It is therefore important for a supervisor to reflect on whether there might be issues that are not being spoken about or are being experienced in the countertransference and not being considered. These might be around sexuality, difference, aggression, hate, envy, love, etc., but can be anything that links to the defensive system of the participants. Thinking the unthinkable is often necessary in supervision and commenting on what is being excluded from the patient/supervisee narrative will make these motifs available for reflective thought in relation to the patient.

Final comment

Our way of being a supervisor with our supervisees can be wide-ranging. There are times to be supportive and empathic; times to be active, informative and educative; times to be reflective, explorative, facilitative, process orientated and interpretive and times to be evaluative and confrontational. But our interventions with our supervisees need to aim to develop understanding and awareness in them about the patient and the processes and dynamics of the therapy. As a supervisor it is therefore important to be aware of how our interactions and interventions affect the supervisee and whether they enable a deeper level of understanding and awareness in them.

Note

1 Hermeneutics is the study of interpretation and meaning.

References

Bion, W.R. (1967) *Second Thoughts*. New York: Aronson.

Bion, W.R. (1970) *Attention and Interpretation*. London: Tavistock Publications Ltd.

Böhm, T. (2002) 'Reflections on psychoanalytic listening'. *Scand. Psychoanal. Rev.* (25) (1):20–26.

Bollas, C. (1991) *The Shadow of the Object*. London: Free Association Books.

Bollas, C. (2002) *Free Association*. Cambridge: Icon Books.

Boston Change Process Study Group (BCPSG) (2013) 'Enactment and the emergence of new relational organization'. *J. Amer. Psychoanal. Assn.* (61): 727–749.

Bravesmith, A. (2008) 'Supervision and imagination'. *J. Anal. Psychol.* (53)(1):101–117.

Britton, R. and Steiner, J. (1994) 'Interpretation: Selected Fact or Overvalued Idea?' *Int. J. Psychoanal.* (75):1069–1078.

Casement, P. (1985) *On Learning from the Patient*. London: Tavistock Publications.

Casement, P. (1990) *Further Learning From the Patient*. London: Routledge.

Crawford, S. (2005) 'Free association and supervision'. Driver, C. and Martin, E. (eds.) *Supervision and the Analytic Attitude*. London: Whurr.

Driver, C. (2005) 'Language and interpretation in supervision'. Driver, C. and Martin, E. (eds.) *Supervision and the Analytic Attitude*. London: Whurr.

Driver, C. (2020) *The Self and the Quintessence*. London and New York: Routledge.

Fonagy, P., Bateman, A. and Luyten, P. (2012) 'Introduction'. Bateman, A. and Fonagy, P. (eds.) *Handbook of Mentalizing in Mental Health Practice. First Edition*. Washington: American Psychiatric Association Publishing.

Fonagy, P. and Bateman, A.W. (2019) 'Introduction'. Bateman, A. and Fonagy, P. (eds.) *Handbook of Mentalizing in Mental Health Practice.* 2nd edition. Washington: American Psychiatric Association Publishing.

Gabbard, G. (2000) 'What can neuroscience teach us about transference?' *Can. J. Psychoanal.* (9):1–18.

Gabbard, G. and Westen, D. (2003) 'Rethinking therapeutic action'. *Int. J. Psychoanal.* (84) (4):823–841.

Gee, H. (1996) 'Developing insight through supervision. Relating, then defining'. *J. Anal. Psychol.* (41) (4):529–552.

Greenson, R.R. (1981) *The Technique and Practice of Psychoanalysis.* London: Hogarth Press.

Jacobs, D., David, P. and Meyer, D.J. (1995) *The Supervisory Encounter.* New Haven and London: Yale University.

Hawkins, P and Shohet, R. (2002) *Supervision in the Helping Professions,* 2nd edition. Buckingham and Philadelphia: Open University Press.

Jung, C.G (1911–12/1952) 'Two kinds of thinking'. *Symbols of Transformation. CW5.* London and Henley: Routledge & Kegan Paul. 1981.

Kernberg, O.F. (2010) 'Psychoanalytic supervision: The supervisor's tasks'. *Psychoanal. Q.* (79) (3):603–627.

Kris, A. (1996) *Free Association: Method and Process.* London: Karnac Books.

Martin, E. (2002) 'Listening to the absent patient'. Driver, C. and Martin, E. (eds.) *Supervising Psychotherapy.* London: Sage Publications.

Mattinson, J. (1997) *The Deadly Equal Triangle.* London: Tavistock Marital Studies Institute.

Nagell, W., Steinmetzer, L., Fissabre, U. and Spilski, J. (2014) 'Research into the relationship experience in supervision and its influence on the psychoanalytical identity formation of candidate trainees'. *Psychoanal. Inq.* (34) (6):554–583.

Ogden, T.H. (1999) *Reverie and Interpretation.* London: Karnac Books.

Ogden, T. (2005) 'On psychoanalytic supervision'. *Int. J. Psychoanal.* (86) (5):1265–1280.

Pally, R. (2003) *The Mind-Brain Relationship.* London: Karnac.

Piaget, J. (1958) *The Development of Thought: Equilibration of Cognitive Structures.* New York: Viking.

Schore, A.N. (2012) 'The right brain implicit self lies at the core of psychoanalysis'. *The Science of the Art of Psychotherapy.* New York and London: W.W. Norton & Co., Ltd

Steele, R.S. (1979) 'Psychoanalysis and hermeneutics'. *Int. Rev. Psycho-Anal.* (6): 389.

Stern, D.N., *et al.* (1998) 'Non-interpretive mechanisms in psychoanalytic therapy: The 'something more' than interpretation. [The Process of Change Study Group]'. *Int. J. PsychoAnal.* (79): 903–921.

Stern, D.N. (2004) *The Present Moment in Psychotherapy and Everyday Life.* New York, NY: Norton.

Szecsödy, I. (1990) *The Learning Process in Psychotherapy Supervision.* Stockholm: Department of Psychiatry, Karolinska Institutet, St Gorans Hospital.

Szecsödy, I. (1997) '(How) is learning possible in supervision?' Martindale, B.*et al.* (eds.) *Supervision and its Vicissitudes.* London: Karnac Books.

Vygotsky, L. (2002) *Thought and Language.* Cambridge, MA and London: The MIT Press.

Westen, D. and Gabbard, G. (2002a) 'Developments in cognitive neuroscience. I. Conflict, compromise, and connectionism'. *J. Amer. Psychoanal. Assn.* (50) (1):53–98.

Westen, D. and Gabbard, G. (2002b) 'Developments in cognitive neuroscience. II. Implications for theories of transference'. *J. Amer. Psychoanal. Assn.* (50) (1):99–134.

Winnicott, D.W. (1979) *The Maturational Processes and the Facilitating Environment.* London: The Hogarth Press.

Winnicott, D.W. (1980) *Playing and Reality.* Harmondsworth: Penguin Books.

Yerushalmi, H. (2018) 'Loneliness, closeness and shared responsibility in supervision'. *Am. J. Psychoanal.* (78) (3):231–246.

Yerushalmi, H. (2024a) 'Future developments in psychoanalytic supervision'. *Psychodynamic Practice* (30) (1):19–29.

Yerushalmi, H. (2024b) 'On solidarity and generosity in supervision'. *Psychodynamic Practice* (30) (3–4):245–254.

Yorke, V. (2005) 'Bion's 'vertex' as a supervisory object'. Driver, C. and Martin, E. (eds.) *Supervision and the Analytic Attitude.* London: Whurr.

Zachrisson, A. (2011) 'Dynamics of psychoanalytic supervision: A heuristic model'. *Int. J. Psychoanal.* (92) (4):943–961.

Chapter 7

Evaluation and assessment in supervision[1]

Evaluation and assessment in supervision is essential in identifying, discerning and evaluating the issues that are being brought into supervision and what and who they belong to. At one level it is about ascertaining and appraising the patient material and the patient's psychopathology and suitability for treatment. At another it is about the appraisal and assessment of the supervisee's capacities, especially within a training setting, and ultimately, their fitness to practice. However, assessment is also about those small, everyday reflections by which the supervisor determines what dynamics and processes are being brought into the supervisory relationship, what they communicate about the patient and the patient's internal world and what they highlight in terms of the learning needs of the supervisee. At a micro level, assessment in supervision is about identifying and determining the work that is emerging with the patient. At a macro level it is about assessing the clinical needs of the patient and the training needs and competencies of the supervisee. Both are an essential part of the supervisor's role.

Identifying the factors to assess in supervision

All aspects of the clinical rhombus (Ekstein and Wallerstein, 1958) and the supervisory matrix (Perry, 2003) impact on the dynamics of supervision and affect and influence the supervisory relationship and the supervisory process. A lack of understanding and assessment of these factors makes it hard to distinguish what is emerging from the patient material, what belongs to the supervisee

DOI: 10.4324/9781003496137-7

and their learning needs, what might belong to the supervisor and what belongs to the context. A supervisor therefore needs to develop the capacity to evaluate and assess the factors involved in the supervisory relationship and what they emerge from so that they can be addressed and worked with. To not do so risks collusion and the danger that key factors are unconsciously enacted, ignored or remain unconscious.

For the supervisor the processes of assessment in supervision requires an ability to discern, evaluate, explore and consider a range of factors including:

- the patient material, the patient's psychopathology and suitability for treatment or referral to other resources
- the supervisee's needs and capabilities, especially within a training setting
- the supervisee's presentation and conscious and unconscious communications
- the conscious and unconscious dynamics between the supervisor and the supervisee and its possible informational value in relation to the patient
- unconscious dynamics from the supervisor's personal material
- organisational issues and their impact on the supervisee and the patient
- fitness to practice issues.

Assessing the patient

To understand the patient requires the evaluation, appraisal and processing of the patient's story as well as the patient's experience so as to build up an hypothesis of how their internal world has evolved and been structured by their life experience. To achieve this understanding by the therapist and supervisor requires a framework from which to formulate an hypothesis about the patient's internal world.

Hinshelwood (1991) comments 'clinical material is best approached as *pictures of relationships with objects*' (p.167), and that formulations and hypotheses are needed in order to create a picture of the internal world of the patient. Hinshelwood (1991) proposes 'three areas of object relationships' (p.167), which he keeps in mind when listening to a patient's story and which provides one way of structuring the information (conscious and unconscious), which a patient presents. He considers the following:

a the current life situation *and patterns of relationships.*
b the infantile object-relations, as described in the patient's history, or hypothesised from what is known.
c the relationship with the assessor which, to all intents and purposes, is the beginning of the transference.

(Hinshelwood, 1991:p.167)

Hinshelwood's criteria enables an assessment of the patient and a way of understanding the issues that the patient is bringing, consciously and unconsciously, to the therapeutic encounter and also to the supervisory one. However, our range of psychoanalytic and psychodynamic theories all provide frameworks from which to assess the patient material and in 2006 The Psychodynamic Diagnostic Manual (PDM Task Force, 2006) was produced to provide one way of evaluating a patient and their problems based on criteria such as personality patterns, mental functioning, symptoms and affects. Whatever conceptualisations we use the aim is to understand the patient, their internal world, their patterns of relating and how this impacts on their life and relationships, including the therapeutic one. To do this, either as a therapist or as a supervisor, we need to employ an analytic attitude that thinks, reflects, questions and explores why the patient is struggling with their problems now and what the issues might relate to. Perry (2003) aptly describes the complexity of supervision as 'entering into the labyrinth' (p.187) in which the supervisor is an explorer, with the supervisee, in identifying and assessing the patient's material and generating a formulation in terms of the patient's presenting problem and the dynamics of their internal world.

    Assessment of the patient material is therefore about identifying the issues that the patient brings, including transference and countertransference, so as to enable the development of the work of the supervisee with their patient. This is important so as to determine the needs of the patient and develop an awareness of what is being projected into the supervisory relationship from them. This helps distinguish between the patient material and other aspects of the clinical rhombus affecting the supervisory dynamic.

Assessment of the supervisee

Evaluation and assessment of supervisees is part of the role of the supervisor but can present both professional and personal challenges. Psychotherapists are often drawn to clinical work through a desire to 'help' and 'heal' (Banks, 2002:p.23) and experienced practitioners often move into becoming supervisors to enable others to develop their clinical work. The danger is that the desire to help and heal can lead to a caring preoccupation and a collusive pairing in which there is no critical or objective position from which to consider and assess the work of the supervisee. Assessment of a supervisee requires taking up a more critical position from which to assess. Assessment disturbs yet informs because it takes us out of the comfort zone of standing alongside the supervisee and places us in the arena of criteria and critique. It also leaves the supervisor as the potential recipient of negative transference, which can be difficult for supervisor and supervisee alike and may activate primitive feelings in both parties. Assessment therefore requires a supervisor to find their own sense of agency and authority in relation to the requirements of a training and the profession and to develop the capacity to empathically hold and challenge as well as confront the difficulties or shortcomings of the supervisee.

For a supervisor this involves being able to maintain a reflective ego and benign superego so that the issues in relation to the supervisee can be processed, addressed and understood. The danger occurs when a supervisor acts from a persecutory superego, and a paranoid-schizoid authoritarian position, rather than an authoritative perspective based in the depressive position (Obholzer, 2006), which can tolerate and accept the good enough (Driver, 2019:p.167). As Stockwell (2005) comments, 'a healthy superego is flexible and adaptive. It is firm and giving, enabling supervisors to assert authority and to praise' (p.92). Authority and assessment therefore requires a benign superego within the supervisor so that they can work creatively, and in an ego related way, to keep communication and dialogue open with the supervisee.

This is one of the challenges of being a supervisor because it requires being able to hold a dual role in relation to the supervisory work and the supervisee. On the one hand, the supervisor needs to work with the supervisee to enable them to assess and explore the presenting issues of the patient as well process countertransference, transference and unconscious communications. On the other hand the supervisor needs to hold an objective attitude in relation to the work of the supervisee in order to evaluate the skills, competencies and abilities, or lack of, in the supervisee and to discuss this with them so as to enable the supervisee to identify the areas they need to develop. Assessment in supervision therefore requires an understanding of assessment criteria and clinical competencies as well as an understanding of how to work with these in a way that is, hopefully, creative for both the supervisee and the clinical work.

Having criteria based on competencies enables the supervisor to objectively identify the competencies and learning needs of the supervisee (see Chapter 5) in relation to the criteria of the training and the profession. Tuckett (2005) comments that using competencies 'can help us move from making global judgements based on implicit criteria towards making specific transparent judgements backed by examples' (p.44). This ensures that assessment and evaluation is objective and not subjectively skewed by the supervisor's own transference to the supervisee. The following issues are helpful to consider in relation to the work of the supervisee:

- The supervisee's manner of relating to the supervisor e.g., dependent, defensive, autonomous, reflective etc.
- The supervisee's manner of relating to the patient e.g., empathic, reflective, insightful, critical, defensive, etc.
- Ability to use theory to form hypotheses about the patient.
- Capacity for independent thinking, reflection and processing.
- Capacity to understand transference, countertransference and unconscious processes.
- Ability to interpret appropriately.
- Capacity to use the self in relation to the patient.
- Open to learning or resistant to learning.

- Capacity to use their internal supervisor (Casement 1985).
- Ability to create and maintain appropriate boundaries in their work and work ethically.

Körner (2002) defines knowledge, technical skills and an analytic attitude as the key criteria in the training of psychoanalytic and psychodynamic practitioners. Kernberg (2010) comments that these three aspects of supervisee development provide a basis for a realistic evaluation of a supervisee's progress but that such an evaluation 'must be shared fully and openly with the supervisee, and the supervisor must remain open to the supervisee's reactions to the supervisor's views' (p.625). Kernberg (2010) also considers that evaluation needs to be an ongoing process so that the supervisee is aware of the areas that they need to develop. In addition, practitioner development and competency can only be achieved over of time. Expecting a trainee in their first year of clinical work to conceptualise and process countertransference phenomena or the manifestations of the reflection process within supervision might be unrealistic but would be something one would expect from a qualified or experienced practitioner. As Dreifuss (1982) comments 'if we assess progress in supervision, we have first to evaluate the supervisee at the beginning of supervision and then assess progress after a period of time and/or hours of supervision' (p.108). Kernberg (2010) states something similar and observes that 'over time, it will become clear to what extent the trainee is developing his or her own frame of reference and integrating knowledge received from the supervisor' (p.624). The supervisory equation in relation to the assessment of the supervisee therefore needs to measure criteria against time, and the passage of time needs to indicate development in relation to the criteria.

Assessment, the supervisee and the patient

Criteria in relation to supervisee competency is only one factor to consider because clinical and supervisory work is always vulnerable to the most important variable and that is the patient. A practitioner may be highly experienced and competent, have a thorough understanding of theory, defences, transference, countertransference and unconscious processes and yet be stuck in their work because the patient is defended against knowing and cannot internalise and integrate their projections. The supervisor is therefore presented with the challenge of how to assess and identify what is happening in the work in terms of what belongs to the patient, what belongs to the supervisee and what is being experienced in the supervision as an interaction of the two via parallel process (Ekstein and Wallerstein, 1958).

For example, Maria presented her patient Jane in supervision. Maria poured out the details of the session and of how Jane talked about her week, the problems she was facing at work and the problems with her boyfriend. Throughout the presentation Maria asked the supervisor what she should say to Jane and what she should do to help her with the difficulties she was facing. Initially the supervisor found herself responding by telling Maria what to say and giving her ideas about what was going on. However, the supervisor also began to feel concerned by Maria's constant questions, her dependency and her lack of ability to think and reflect. She began to wonder about Maria's capabilities as a therapist.

Noting her negative responses to Maria's work the supervisor began to think about her countertransference to Maria's presentation and her sense of Maria's dependency. Whilst reflecting on this the supervisor suggested to Maria that they think more about the patient's early relationships so that they might begin to make sense of the transference and Jane's patterns of relationships. Maria began to describe Jane's background and history and realised, as she did so, the extent of Jane's problems around separation from an overprotective mother and her dependency on others. As consideration of this progressed, the supervisor reflected to herself that in the presentations of this patient Maria had also become very dependant and helpless and that what was being experienced in the supervision was a powerful parallel process of the patient's pathology. The supervisor commented to Maria that dependency and helplessness seemed to have become a powerful component of Jane's transference to Maria and that this had also been reflected in the supervision. Maria was able to reflect on this and commented on how difficult it was to feel how dependent Jane was on her.

This example contains a number of overlapping dynamics. Jane, the patient, brought into the therapeutic relationship her patterns of relating, which revealed a dynamic of dependency, helplessness and anxiety. Maria, as a relatively new practitioner, was vulnerable to anxiety and wanted to be accepted. As a result, in supervision Maria's presentation of the work with Jane not only reflected the patient's helplessness, dependency and transference issues but also Maria's anxiety of wanting to do things right. If the supervisor had acted on her critical responses it would have inappropriately placed the focus onto Maria's competency and overlooked the impact on the supervisory dynamic of the patient material. Only time would tell if issues of dependency and helplessness in Maria was a transitory phase in relation to the work with Jane or an ongoing problem.

Determining the factors that are affecting the supervisory process is vital so as to ensure that one aspect of it does not become a scapegoat in relation to the impact of the others. Also, it is difficult to assess the work of a supervisee on one patient alone because different dynamics may or will emerge with different patients. Assessment, evaluation, differentiation and identification of what belongs to whom is therefore a key responsibility of a supervisor and requires a supervisor to consider all the dimensions of the supervisory dynamic within the clinical rhombus.

Assessment in supervision: an open or closed system?

Criteria are helpful in identifying what needs to be looked for but they do not identify the processes through which assessment takes place. One of the challenges in relation to the supervisee is how to integrate assessment into the dialogue of the supervisory relationship. In the past this was often carried out by the supervisor writing a report about the supervisee, which was not seen by the supervisee. This led to the invidious- and paranoia-producing situation in which the supervisee had to wait until the verdict came from the training committee or equivalent to discover the outcome of the supervisor's assessment. What was avoided in this procedure was the delicate and sometimes difficult and painful process of giving feedback to the supervisee in person.

The challenge in giving feedback is that it can break up the good feeling between the supervisor and supervisee, open up the negative transference and mean both supervisor and supervisee facing what is feared, disowned and possibly shame inducing. The obstacles to the processes of assessment for the supervisee, which Plaut (1982) identified, were 'fear of the supervisor's power, fear of losing the patient, fear of ignorance' (p.106) and submission to, or denial of, the supervisor's power. The challenge for the supervisor is holding the tension between being perceived as, or becoming, the critical and powerful other, whilst also finding the authority to identify issues with the supervisee that are difficult to acknowledge. In an open assessment this can create defensive and shame-inducing (Martin 2005) dynamics in both parties, but it can also allow for the potential for insight, learning and development. In addition a 'supervisor's avoidance of fully honest criticism puts programme authorities (*and organisations*) in a difficult position' (McWilliams, 2021:p.125).

In an open and transparent system of supervisee evaluation and assessment, consideration of the learning needs of the supervisee can be both productive and creative. When the learning needs and areas of competence, or lack of, can be identified with the supervisee, it enables the supervisee to take active steps to tackle the problems. The advantage of open assessment is that it both confronts and values the adult ego of both parties whilst simultaneously containing the struggle with the transference to the supervisor and the regressive pull in the supervisee. If this can be held sensitively the defences within both supervisor and supervisee can be minimised and a productive dialogue generated. It is when the supervisor's superego becomes persecutory, or is experienced in that way, or the supervisee is resistant to learning that the process can become stuck and requires insight in one or both parties to identify what is being struggled with. A closed assessment system, in which the supervisee is kept in the dark about what they are required to develop, often results in anger and misunderstandings which are counterproductive to the learning and development of the supervisee.

When problems persist however, it is the supervisor's task to identify when the supervisee's work is not fit for task and when there is a fitness to practice issue. Giving negative feedback is never easy but essential for the development of the supervisee and to ensure the supervisee's development to a competent and ethical practitioner. McWilliams (2021) comments that when giving negative feedback, 'we need to keep all our comments, especially our negative evaluations, tied tightly to the supervisee's behaviour rather than giving our diagnostic impressions of the supervisee. Secondly, we need to share our evaluative thoughts (tactfully) with our supervisees' (p.155). McWilliams goes on to point out that nothing of an evaluative nature in the trainee's 'formal training should be a surprise' (p.155). She stresses the importance of ongoing feedback to the supervisee so that they are aware of the areas that they need to work on and develop.

Evaluation and assessment is an ongoing activity for the supervisor especially with trainees and candidates in training. However, it is also about fitness to practice in terms of clinical and ethical criteria (see Chapter 8) and to confront, if necessary, the difficult, but important, task of bringing someone's training or clinical work to an end in order to protect the patient.

The supervisor and the supervisee

Another aspect of the supervisory relationship that needs to be considered and evaluated by the supervisor is that between themselves and the supervisee. It is vital that a supervisor reflects on what they bring to the process in terms of their transference issues, their subjective assumptions and internal prejudices (Stimmel, 1995). Evaluation by the supervisor of their own internal dynamics is crucial so as to ascertain what might be mixed into the process. Key factors to consider in relation to this are the,

- relationship between the supervisor and the supervisee(s)
- impact of the patient on the supervisory process and possible parallel processes
- supervisor's dumb spots or blind spots
- supervisor's countertransference
- impact of the triangular relationship of patient, supervisee and supervisor
- impact of the organisation / training.

This requires a supervisor to utilise their observational capacity and internal reflections so that they can ponder on and consider the experiences that they are involved in with their supervisee and identify what or who they belong to (see also Chapter 5).

The impact of organisational issues

In addition to assessing and working with clinical issues in relation to the patient and the learning needs of the supervisee a supervisor also needs to assess and consider the impact of organisational issues on the dynamics of supervision. In one organisation the dynamics of the supervision always changed at the time of the year when the trainees were being assessed in their training. The trainees/supervisees would frequently present patient material which contained issues relating to a critical superego, shame and criticism. Such material unconsciously created a powerful parallel process of critical others, which belonged to both the patient and the supervisee but was prompted by the organisation's demands. When such dynamics arise it is important for a supervisor to remain focused on the patient's issues but be simultaneously aware of the related dynamics and anxiety in the supervisee.

The dynamics of the organisation inevitably impact on the clinical and supervisory work and as a result it is important to take into account,

- the nature of the organisation and the nature of the patient/ client group that are being brought into the supervision
- the demands of the organisation on the supervisor and the supervisee
- whether the organisation provides a safe frame for the clinical work and the supervision
- whether the organisation understands the needs of the patient/ client group and the needs of the therapists
- whether it provides initial assessments and has psychiatric backing
- whether it is a training organisation and/or a clinical service.

All of these factors have an impact on the supervisory process and can affect the clinical work, the supervisory relationship and the supervisory encounter. Assessment and evaluation of the impact of organisational issues on the dynamics of supervision process is vital so as to clarify the issues involved.

Final comment

Ekstein and Wallerstein's (1958) model of the clinical rhombus illustrates the manner in which the overlapping conscious and unconscious dynamics of supervisor, supervisee, patient and the context influence and impact on the clinical work. Without evaluation and assessment of the factors involved, and the conscious and unconscious communications within the supervisory relationship, it can be hard to distinguish what is emerging from the patient material and what belongs to the supervisee and their learning needs. Assessing and understanding all of the relational interactive dynamics is a challenge for the supervisor because it requires separation and assessment in order to identify and clarify the factors involved so that they can be addressed and worked with. To not do so risks collusion and the danger that key factors are unconsciously enacted, ignored or remain unconscious. Assessment of the elements and constituents of the supervisory relationship provides a process from which to understand the aetiology of the complex set of components within the supervisory dynamic and identification of the tasks in relation to the patient and the supervisee.

Evaluation and assessment brings in issues of appraisal and differentiation in relation to the work between the patient, the therapist/supervisee and supervisor. It also involves identifying any organisational dynamics caught up in the supervisory and clinical process. A supervisor is gate-keeper, container, educator, explorer and artist in relation to both patient and supervisee. The processes of evaluation and assessment are to ensure that understanding about the patient and the therapeutic work is achieved and the clinical work of the supervisee developed. Assessment can therefore be a creative process, but it is also a challenging one in relation to the supervisory relationship, the work of the supervisee and the development of ethical good practice. The aim is to ensure understanding and awareness of the factors that coalesce within the supervisory relationship and ensure that the supervisee is an effective and safe container and fit for the task of the work with the patient.

Note

1 A version of this chapter was previously published in the *British Journal of Psychotherapy*. Driver, C (2008) 'Assessment in supervision: An analytic perspective'. *Brit. J. Psychother.* (24)(3):328–342.

References

Banks, M. (2002) 'The transition from therapist to supervisor'. Driver, C. and Martin, E. (Eds) *Supervising Psychotherapy*. London: Sage.

Casement, P. (1985) *On Learning from the Patient*. London: Tavistock Publications.

Dreifuss, G. (1982) 'Symposium: How Do I assess progress in supervision?'. *J. of Anal. Psychol.* (27):107–110.

Driver, C. (2008) 'Assessment in supervision: An analytic perspective'. *Brit. J. of Psychother.* (24)(3).

Driver, C. (2019) 'The superego as a significant factor in clinical training'. Harding, C. (ed.) *Dissecting the Superego*. London: Routledge.

Ekstein, R. and Wallerstein, R.S. (1958) *The Teaching and Learning of Psychotherapy*. Madison Connecticut: International Universities Press, Inc.

Hinshelwood, R.D. (1991) 'Psychodynamic formulation in assessment for psychotherapy'. *Brit. J. of Psychother.* (8)(2):166–174.

Kernberg, O.F. (2010) 'Psychoanalytic supervision: The supervisor's tasks'. *Psychoanal. Q.* (79)(3):603–627.

Körner, J. (2002) 'The didactics of psychoanalytic education'. *Int. J. PsychoAnal.*, (83):1395–1405.

Martin, E. (2005) 'Shame in supervision'. Driver, C. and Martin, E. (eds.) *Supervision and the Analytic Attitude*. London: Whurr.

McWilliams, N. (2021) *Psychoanalytic Supervision*. New York and London: The Guilford Press.

Obholzer, A. (2006) 'Authority, power and leadership: contributions from group relations training'. Obholzer, A. and Zagier Roberts, V. (eds.) *The Unconscious at Work; Individual and Organisational Stress in Human Services*. Hove, England, Routledge.

PDM Task Force (2006) *Psychodynamic Diagnostic Manual*. Silver Spring, MD; Alliance of Psychoanalytic Organizations.

Perry, C. (2003) 'Into the labyrinth: A developing approach to supervision'. Wiener, J., Mizen, R. and Duckham, J. (eds.) *Supervision and*

Being Supervised: A Practice in Search of a Theory. Basingstoke: Palgrave Macmillan.

Plaut, F. (1982) 'Symposium: How do I assess Progress in supervision?' *J. of Anal. Psychol.* (27):105–107.

Stimmel, B. (1995) 'Resistance to awareness of the supervisor's transference with special reference to the parallel process'. *Int. J. Psycho-anal.* (76)(6):609–618.

Stockwell, R. (2005) 'The ego and superego in supervision'. Driver, C. and Martin, E. (Eds) *Supervision and the Analytic Attitude.* London: Whurr.

Tuckett, D. (2005) 'Does anything go? Towards a framework for the more transparent assessment of psychoanalytic competence'. *The Int. J. Psychoanal.* (86)(1):31–49.

Chapter 8

Ethics and professional standards in supervision

Becoming and being a supervisor involves taking on ethical responsibility and professional authority in relation to the supervisee and their work. This requires supervisors to abide by the same professional standards, criteria of confidentiality and codes of ethics as those of their professional memberships as analysts, psychotherapists and supervisors and the Code of Ethics and Practice of their registering body. But ethical practice goes beyond rules and codes, it requires an ethical attitude within the practitioner and 'addressing and protecting the internal world of the patient' (Martin, 2003:p.136) and the supervisee. So, although Codes of Ethics provide the external rules and state some absolute no go areas such as sexual enactments or financial exploitation, they are only part of what it means to work ethically. Many issues are more subtle and require careful consideration between the supervisor and supervisee in order to make informed judgements appropriate to the circumstances.

Ethics and an ethical attitude

Working ethically requires an ethical attitude in relation to the patient and the supervisee. An ethical attitude entails integrity and holding a 'third position, a mental and emotional ethical space where the subjective and the objective, the ethical and the unethical can be considered' (Wiener, 2001:p.431). This 'third position' (Solomon, 2001) and ethical attitude involves maintaining the tension between conflicting thoughts and actions and considering

DOI: 10.4324/9781003496137-8

and exploring such conflicts with integrity in relation to the well-being of the patient and the supervisee. McFarland Solomon and Twyman (2003) examine this in detail and McFarland Solomon (2007) considers that an 'analytic attitude is an ethical attitude, and that the ethical attitude is a developmental achievement, and as such it may reach beyond the depressive position' (p.443). This is because an ethical attitude involves dealing with uncertainty and struggling with our inner world and the conscious and unconscious eddies and flows of our emotions, attitudes and instincts. It also 'involves doubt and uncertainty. There are often no clear answers, but rather dilemmas with which analysts need to grapple' (Allphin, 2005:p.452).

Examining potential ethical dilemmas within psychoanalytic and psychodynamic work therefore requires diligence and an ethical attitude in the supervisor and in their exploration with their supervisees. In addition, an ethical attitude and an openness to engaging with issues around equality, diversity, inclusion and intersectionality are important. Supervisors also need to hold an ethical attitude in relation to their own work, which may require a consultation with a colleague. Ethical challenges are best discussed. Secrets lead to the danger of oversights or enactments. In addition, a central aspect of ethical practice 'is passing on to the next generation of practitioners the moral sensibilities that inform psychotherapy' (McWilliams, 2021:p.109). In supervision we aim to work in an ego-related way but 'we should not underestimate the power of the unconscious and, when we are in its grip, even the simplest of rules may provide the essential ingredient to help the supervisee, *and supervisor* [1], maintain an ethical position' (Gee, 2003:p.164). Codes of Ethics and an ethical attitude that is open to exploration and finding an ethical solution are vital in relation to all aspects of supervisory work.

Ethics and the patient

In supervision, ethical standards and responsibilities relate to the supervisee and the patient and also the tricky area surrounding clinical responsibility. Sometimes the supervisor will need to be active in supporting the supervisee to encourage a patient to contact medical services when suicidal ideation is prevalent or when mental health issues become serious. Or explore and respond to issues related to concerns such as safeguarding or terrorism. In the United Kingdom this is a requirement and organisations offering counselling or therapy must have a safeguarding policy and a safeguarding lead who can be consulted if such situations arise. But such issues also require the supervisor to help the supervisee consider how to speak to the patient about them or how to inform the patient that they (the therapist) will need to speak to other services about the issues raised. This might entail breaking confidentiality and so requires detailed and difficult discussions between the supervisor and the supervisee and, ultimately, the patient.

However, clinical responsibility is a difficult area for a supervisor and the process of supervision. A supervisor only hears about the issues that a patient brings after the patient's session with the therapist/supervisee. Sadly, sometimes information will be received of suicide after it has happened because the patient has not spoken about suicidal thoughts in the therapy or, worryingly, the supervisee has not brought such concerns to supervision. Sometimes concerns about suicide or other major issues require a break in the supervisory boundary so that a supervisee can contact the supervisor in-between sessions. When such concerns are expressed in supervision about a patient it is useful for a supervisor to make a note of actions suggested, or taken, by themselves or the supervisee. This will provide important evidence or information in the event of an investigation or inquest. Kernberg (2010) is of the opinion that 'the ideal situation between supervisor and supervisee is one in which both parties are clear that the supervisee ultimately carries this (clinical) responsibility' (p.616) for the patient. But, within an organisation, such as a training or clinical service, the 'ultimate responsibility may lie with the institution' (ibid) and the supervisee, 'under certain circumstances, may have to comply with the supervisor's instructions' (p.616). Issues of clinical responsibility therefore need to be clearly communicated, but painful and difficult decisions often still need to be made about the supervisee or the work with the patient.

Although a supervisor will only hear about a patient after a session, any information that raises ethical and clinical concerns requires careful and open discussion with the supervisee in order to help them understand the issues involved and how to respond. It is therefore vital that a supervisor holds an ethical attitude in relation to the patient and the supervisee and works with the supervisee to develop their ethical attitude. However sometimes situations arise in supervision in relation to the patient or the supervisee when a supervisor has to consider 'when it is time to manage rather than supervise' (Martin, 2003:p.146).

Ethics and the supervisee

The role of the supervisor in relation to the supervisee is complex because it relates to their development as clinicians, assessment in training and fitness to practice issues. This gives a supervisor power in relation to the supervisee but also responsibilities, both of which require an ethical attitude and a benign authority in relation to the supervisee's work. Decisions about training competencies, trainee assessments or fitness to practice issues need to link to Codes of Ethics and evidence in relation to such requirements are essential.

Ethical challenges in relation to a supervisee are difficult and painful especially when decisions and actions have to be taken in relation to the moral and ethical codes of the profession. Blatant acting out or a serious breach of ethical codes will normally also involve an ethics committee and may require a supervisor to work with the supervisee to end their clinical work with their patients and, if a trainee, end their training. As McWilliams (2021) comments, the supervisor's ethical responsibility 'is to protect the public against clinicians who are … incompetent or corrupt' (p.110) and whose work is inappropriate. However many professional or clinical concerns are less clear cut and belong to what Primo Levi (Primo Levi quoted in Abramovitch, 2007) called a 'grey zone' where 'boundaries between good and bad are unclear' (p.449). This is where an ethical attitude is vital in terms of holding and considering both the positive and negative aspects of a supervisee's work and the balance between the two. In such situations the supervisor's ongoing evidence of the supervisee's clinical work is vital in relation to the competences and fitness to practice requirements of the profession. In addition consultation with another supervisor, or clinical team, is useful in order to discuss the issues of concern because this enables a wider perspective to be considered and a decision reached based on a consensus. Within an organisation such a process is achievable but the danger in private practice is that a supervisor holds the power and anxiety of being responsible for any decision. This is where an ethical danger lies because being the sole authority when making ethical decisions can lead to a mis-use of power and an entrenched position that is closed to reflection. Again this is where discussion with another supervisor about concerns about a supervisee or a patient are important. Discussion reflects an ethical attitude and alleviates the pressure on a supervisor in relation to any ethical and clinical decisions that may need to be made.

The assessment role of a supervisor in relation to a trainee can also be a challenge (see Chapter 7). One of the differences between being an analyst and being a supervisor 'is that supervisors are often asked to make value judgements on their supervisee's work' (Martin, 2003:p.141). Holding such a role requires the supervisor to make judgements and decisions about the supervisee based on the competencies required by the training. In such situations, it is important for the supervisor to discuss their view of the supervisee's work with others and consider whether their point of view is based on sound evidence and an objective perspective.

Ending the work of a supervisee is never easy; it can stir up anxiety in the supervisor and negative transference issues from the supervisee. It is important, however, to keep in mind that it is the well-being of the patient that is the focus and that when a 'supervisee's work is not fit for task or when there is a fitness to practice issue' this needs to be openly discussed with the supervisee to 'help them see what needs to be considered or to end their clinical work in order to protect the patient or, perhaps, the supervisee' (Driver, 2023:p.10). Such processes are not straightforward and can be challenging so having collegial or supervisory support as a supervisor is helpful when such issues arise.

Another role of the supervisor concerns the well-being of the supervisee and their capacity to work effectively. When supervising clinical work where issues of trauma, violence, death, abuse, rape, sexual exploitation, etc., are the main focus issues of vicarious traumatisation need to be considered in relation to both supervisee and supervisor. This is especially important when supervising in organisations that focus on specific and traumatic issues. In such situations the supervisor needs to consider whether the supervisee is becoming overwhelmed by the issues and on the edge of burn-out and discuss this with them. Supervisors also need to consider whether they are becoming traumatised by the material or are themselves on the edge of burn-out.

Issue may also arise in relation to the personal life of the supervisee. Bereavement, illness, pregnancy, birth, divorce, etc., all have a psychological impact that may take the focus of the supervisee away from the patient and onto their own needs. In such situations the supervisor may need to help the supervisee to come to the decision to pause their work so as to give themselves time and space for their own emotions and deal with their own issues. This also brings up the clinical and ethical issue about what to tell the patient. This requires careful and sensitive evaluation in relation to each patient. McWilliams (2021) comments that 'therapy depends on honesty. We need to frankly inform our clients and give them some choice about whether to continue treatment or make a termination plan' (p.113). However, everyone deals with such situations differently and there is no absolute rule about this, but it is helpful for the supervisor to explore such issues with a supervisee so as to find out what is in the best interest of the supervisee and the patient. Such issues may also affect the supervisor and it is helpful for the supervisor to also consider if they have the inner mental and emotional space to work during difficult periods in their own lives.

Speaking about concerns to a supervisee requires shifting the focus from the patient onto the supervisee for a period of time. This is more straightforward in one-to-one supervision, but is more of a challenge in a group because some of the issues to be explored may be intensely personal for the supervisee or shame-inducing. It is therefore sometimes useful to have one-to-one feedback sessions with each member of a group or, if there are serious concerns about a supervisee's work, to have a one-to-one meeting with the supervisee to discuss the concerns about their work and any fitness to practice issues.

Another ethical issue are boundary overlaps. In a supervision group, for example, there is the potential for the supervisor to be supervising a therapist whose patient is a friend or colleague of another member of the group. One solution is to ask the supervisee who is the friend or colleague of the patient to leave the group whilst the work with that patient is presented. Or, if it is possible, the work of the supervisee with that patient might be taken to supervision with another supervisor. Such boundary issues need careful consideration to ensure that issues around confidentiality and supervisory and clinical boundaries are maintained.

Cultivating an ethical attitude in a supervisee is an intrinsic part of supervisory work. When transference or countertransference issues arise in relation to a patient or a patient is putting pressure on a therapist/supervisee it is often helpful to explore the ethical challenges that are being presented. The real danger is when a supervisee doesn't talk about the challenges of the work because 'secrecy, doing something we would not want to become known, is one of the key warning signals that we are on the slippery slope towards an ethical violation' (Abramovitch, 2007:p.457). Berman (2000) advises that the 'ethical option is to create in supervision a tolerant and attentive atmosphere, which will make it easier for trainees/supervisees to share personal associations and feelings whenever they appear to be potentially relevant to the task in hand' (p.284). It is through reflection with the supervisee that a supervisor mirrors an ethical and analytic attitude in relation to the patient and the issues that they present.

Ethics and the supervisor

The supervisory relationship is not the same as the therapeutic one and with qualified supervisees it is sometimes almost collegial. But a supervisor does have a different role and responsibilities to those of a supervisee and also a different authority. This authority is not about knowledge of theory, although that might form part of their role, it is authority in relation to the development of the work of the supervisee with the patient, transference and counter-transference dynamics, regression and fitness to practice issues. These all link to the evaluation and assessment role of a

supervisor and the need to challenge and confront fitness to practice issues if they arise.

An ethical attitude also relates to the supervisory relationship
and the transference and countertransference of the supervisor to
the supervisee. As commented on earlier in this book (see Chapter
5), a supervisor needs to be mindful of their own transference
responses to a supervisee and be aware that not everything can be
explained by parallel process. For a supervisor a supervisee can, in
the transference, represent a favourite or problem internal object
in relation to the supervisor's history and internal world (Stimmel,
1995). It is also important for a supervisor to be aware of the
power dynamics present in supervision and that in supervision
there is always a power differential. This generates complex
transference issues from supervisee to supervisor because of
dependency issues, learning needs, projections and idealisation.
What we need to be wary of is what Guggenbühl-Craig (1996)
calls the 'power shadow' (p.85) and the danger of considering that
we are right because we are the professional supervisor. Such a
dynamic feeds into the transference and leads to the creation of a
polarisation between the powerful supervisor and the childish
supervisee. This can be destructive because it denies or destroys
the creativity and therapeutic ability of the supervisee and restricts
their development in relation to the work with the patient.

But perhaps the most difficult area is when there is a sexual/
erotic transference from the supervisor to the supervisee or the
supervisee to the supervisor and the danger of enactments. The
challenge of supervision is that it occurs through a relationship,
albeit a professional one, and requires 'emotional engagement'
(Mann, 1997:p.11). Mann identifies that 'from infancy onwards
the erotic brings people into relationship with others' (Mann,
2001:p.68) and that 'in the "real world" it is that very erotic
experience which is one of the most transformational forces in the
life of most individuals' (p.68). However, therapeutic work and
supervision takes place in a world that exists inside and outside of
the real world and also in the realm of fantasy and the unconscious. As a result the erotic can be creative but also destructive.
Guggenbühl-Craig (1996) comments, 'every human relation may
be negative or positive. There is love and hate in every

relationship, a desire to help the other and at the same time to destroy them' (p.60). This has profound implications for both the therapeutic and supervisory relationship because it identifies the conflicting dynamics present when powerful feelings are aroused. Guggenbühl-Craig (1996) goes on to comment in relation to therapeutic work, 'if the relationship is lived out sexually it becomes no longer the vessel in which the healing process takes place, it becomes an end in itself and thus destroys the therapy' (p.63) or the supervision. Enactments by a supervisor in relation to a supervisee breaks the boundaries of the supervisory frame, destroys the focus of the supervisory work and the analytic and ethical attitude in relation to the development of the supervisee and the work with the patient.

When such feelings arise the important step is understanding what they mean in relation to the supervisee and the patient. McWilliams (2021) comments that 'erotic transferences are certainly not inevitable or universal, and they rarely arise in the first few sessions. When they do, they tend to signify not so much desire as an effort to exert power' (p.127). However when they do arise they also need to be reflected on internally by the supervisor as to what they represent. In addition the supervisor needs to consider the difficult, but important question of 'how we are going to consider the erotic but not fall into its seductions, either by blatant acting out ... or a flight from the erotic' (Mann, 2001: p.74). A question we all need to reflect on.

Ethics and the organisational context of supervision

Ethics in relation to the organisational context of supervision is important. Organisations should have their own complaints procedures, equality policies, safeguarding policies and Code of Ethics. There may be times when a supervisor will need to report to the organisation's management concerns about a supervisee or a patient. Throughout, however an ethical attitude is essential. A complaint by a patient or a therapist needs looking into either at supervisory or management level because complaints are seldom straightforward and all aspects need consideration. McWilliams (2021) specifically identifies the issues that can arise in training institutes in terms of power, envy, rivalry and boundary overlaps and the need for an ethical attitude and ethical standards in relation to all aspects of analytic and therapy trainings.

Ethics and the internet

With the growing prevalence of online work, both clinically and for supervision, it is necessary for a supervisor to give ethical consideration to the online presence and social media activities of themselves and their supervisees. The internet is a rich resource, but it can also be used to obtain information that would previously have been confidential. Online information therefore needs to be considered and discussed in terms of ethics and confidentiality.

Anonymity for either supervisor or therapist can no longer be assured and patient, therapist or supervisor all have the potential to find out, or eavesdrop, on the other through posts on social media and online searches. Holiday photos or intimate family or relationship details are easily accessed on open access sites and are best posted on private closed sites. It is therefore important to consider what a supervisor or a supervisee post online or is available as open access on the internet and to discuss 'ground rules for personal safety and comfort ... and self-care' (McWilliams, 2021: p.131) – something that a supervisor also needs to put in place. Care also needs to be taken when a supervisee or supervisor contact each other online via email etc., because the sharing of clinical information should only occur through safe and confidential channels.[2] The same requirement of a confidential and secure online resource applies to seeing supervisees or patients online.

Final comment

Relationships hold the potential for something creative, but also the potential for something destructive. We all hold a dark side that we want to keep hidden, but our ethical attitude and Codes of Ethics provides a container from which to protect ourselves and others. Ethics and an ethical attitude are necessary to protect the patient and the supervisee and ensure that they have a safe, confidential and boundaried space in which to work. Solomon (2001) writes that an ethical attitude should be an intrinsic part of the analyst's and supervisor's self and needs to be based on humaneness and acting humanely toward others in our professional lives as well as in our personal lives. It also requires us to hold an analytic and ethical attitude in relation to our work as clinicians and supervisors. Brodsky (2017) comments that 'ethics is the platform that holds the capacity for analytic thought, and analytic thought is the platform for ethics. The supervision process must combine the two' (p.409). It is also helpful, when ethical issues arise, to have a confidential discussion with another supervisor, an ethics committee or legal representative. Through such discussions the issues can be explored and a decision or way forward reached based on ethical principles.

Holding an ethical and analytic attitude in conjunction with each other is challenging because it requires us to reflect on difficult issues and feelings, deal with ambiguity and paradox and be open to a position that involves embracing a careful and thoughtful ethical stance, but for the development of a safe and contained space for the patient and the supervisee, it is essential.

Notes

1 My insertion.
2 Many online channels are now end-to-end encrypted but this always needs to be checked.

References

Abramovitch, H. (2007) 'Stimulating ethical awareness during training'. *J. Anal. Psychol.* (52)(4):449–461.

Allphin, C. (2005) 'An ethical attitude in the analytic relationship'. *J. Anal. Psychol.* (50)(4):451–468.

Berman, E. (2000) 'Psychoanalytic supervision. The intersubjective development'. *Int. J. Psychoanal.* (81)(2):273–290.

Brodsky, H. (2017) 'Supervision triangles and the attempt to turn a blind eye to them'. *Contemp. Psychoanal.* (53)(3):393–413.

Driver, C. (2023) 'The superego in supervision. Censor, persecutor or protector'. *Psychodynamic Practice.* https://doi.org/10.1080/14753634.2023.2282721.

Gee, H. (2003) 'Boundaries in supervision'. Wiener, J., Mizen, R. and Duckham, J. (eds.) *Supervision and Being Supervised: A Practice in Search of a Theory.* Basingstoke: Palgrave Macmillan.

Guggenbühl-Craig, A. (1996) *Power in the Helping Professions.* Woodstock, CT: Spring Publications, Inc.

Kernberg, O.F. (2010) 'Psychoanalytic supervision: The supervisor's tasks'. *Psychoanal. Q.* (79)(3):603–627.

Mann, D. (1997) *Psychotherapy. An Erotic Relationship. Transference and Countertransference Passions.* London and New York: Routledge.

Mann, D. (2001) 'Erotics and ethics: The passionate dilemmas of the therapeutic couple'. Palmer Barnes, F. and Murdin, L. (eds.) *Values and Ethics in the Practice of Psychotherapy and Counselling.* Buckingham and Philadelphia: Open University.

Martin, E. (2003) 'Problems and ethical issues in supervision'. Wiener, J., Mizen, R. and Duckham, J. (eds.) *Supervision and Being Supervised: A Practice in Search of a Theory.* Basingstoke: Palgrave Macmillan.

McFarland Solomon, H. and Twyman, M. (eds.) (2003) *The Ethical Attitude in Analytic Practice.* London and New York: Free Association Books.

McFarland Solomon, H. (2007) 'The ethics of supervision: developmental and archetypal perspectives'. Petts, A. and Shapley, B. (eds.) *On Supervision. Psychoanalytic and Jungian Perspectives.* London: Karnac.

McWilliams, N. (2021) *Psychoanalytic Supervision.* New York and London: The Guilford Press.

Solomon, H. (2001) 'Origins of the ethical attitude'. *J. Anal. Psychol.* (46)(3):443–454.

Stimmel, B. (1995) 'Resistance to awareness of the supervisor's transference with special reference to the parallel process'. *International Journal of Psycho-analysis* (76)(6):609–618.

Wiener, J. (2001) 'Confidentiality and paradox. The location of ethical space'. *J. Anal. Psychol.* (46)(3):431–442.

Chapter 9

Being a supervisor

Being a supervisor

Becoming a supervisor and developing a supervisory attitude requires managing, reflecting on and processing complexity in relation to the multi-layered and multifaceted dynamics of supervision and the supervisory relationship. Throughout this book links have been made to the concept of the clinical rhombus (Ekstein and Wallerstein, 1958) because this symbolises the inter-relational factors that a supervisor needs to consider in relation to each patient, supervisee and the dynamics of the supervisory process.

Being a supervisor therefore requires additional capacities (Zachrisson, 2011) and competences to those of a psychodynamic or psychoanalytic clinician and the skills, tasks and efficacy of supervision is one that every practitioner needs to consider. Roth and Pilling (2015) consider that 'ultimately, the purpose of supervision should be to enhance client outcomes' (p.5) and, based on their research, they have produced a supervisor competencies framework (Roth and Pilling, 2015) that summarises the range of generic, specific and metacompetences that a supervisor needs to attain. Szecsödy (2014) outlines goals and criteria for training supervisors and Watkins (2014), in his explorations, outlines six 'broad based' competencies in relation to supervision, such as,

1   knowledge about/understanding of psychoanalytic *and psychodynamic* [1] supervision models, methods and interventions, including the dynamics of unconscious processes.

DOI: 10.4324/9781003496137-9

2 knowledge about/skill in attending to matters of ethical, legal, and professional concern (*including gatekeeping in relation to fitness to practice*).
3 knowledge about/skill in managing psychoanalytic supervision relationship processes.
4 knowledge about/skill in conducting psychoanalytic supervisory assessment and evaluation.
5 knowledge about/skill in fostering attention to difference and diversity.
6 openness to/utilization of a self-reflective, self-assessment stance in psychoanalytic *and psychodynamic* supervision.(p.220)

Competences are important because they outline the skills and attitudes required of a supervisor, but becoming a supervisor is also about creating a safe and boundaried space, either in person or online, in which to explore and hold an attitude of mind which is open to learning, discovery and processing with the supervisee about the patient. Becoming a supervisor is a journey of learning and, just as a trainee therapist moves from being self-focused to process-focused (see Chapter 5), development as a supervisor covers the same trajectory. Beginning any new profession brings up questions of how to do it and holding the anxiety of not-knowing because learning and understanding occurs through the gradual integration of theory and practice and an openness to process in order to understand.

Supervision of supervision

Becoming a supervisor requires attaining new skills and internal capacities in relation to understanding the learning needs of the supervisee and the patient issues. Supervision of supervision facilitates this and is certainly vital when taking the first steps of becoming a supervisor but is ongoing supervision of supervision important? Such a question brings into focus the purpose of supervision of supervision. Power (2013) comments that,

The purpose and process of supervision of supervision are similar to those of supervision. The aim is to make some of the unconscious conscious and to facilitate a containing and generative space where the clinician bringing their work is enabled to think more deeply about the dynamics occurring in another relationship.

(p.391)

Supervision of supervision therefore provides a container in which to explore the work with the supervisee and the patient. Supervision of supervision also enables exploration of the inter-relationship between the supervisor, the therapist/supervisee and the patient and creates the potential to 'start something up in the mind of the supervisor about the supervision that can be used to make a creative and meaningful supervisory intervention' (Mander, 2002:p.139). What supervision of supervision also provides is a layer of consultancy and is especially important when difficulties arise in the supervisory relationship, when there is a fitness to practice issue in relation to the supervisee or there are concerns about the patient. When difficulties arise in the supervisory relationship it can be all too easy to fall into the trap of focusing the problem on the supervisee and overlook transference and countertransference dynamics emanating from the patient and/or the supervisor. Seeking another view when such dynamics arise is vital in order to try to unravel what is caught up in the problem and what the issues relate to.

Supervision of supervision is, therefore, not about providing an 'all-knowing' (Gee, 1996) perspective but rather another viewpoint on the issues presented. Supervision of supervision can also add to the complexity of the inter-relational dynamics of supervision and Mander (2002) cautions against the 'unnecessary and unwieldy proliferation of watchdogs *ad infinitum*' (p.132). But, on the other hand, supervision of supervision, or a supervisory consultation, provides another viewpoint and another mind with whom to think and reflect on the issues and concerns arising for the supervisor and their supervision work.

Being a supervisor – final comment

Being a supervisor is a profession in its own right and requires a practitioner to develop new skills and understandings and the capacity to work with a meta-perspective in relation to the work of the supervisee and the supervisee's work with the patient. Being a supervisor is, to use Zachrisson's (2011) phrase, 'a composite craft' (p.957) that 'requires skills, procedural knowledge, knowledge of concepts and theories and an analytic attitude and ways of thinking and reflecting' (p.948). It is a complex task that requires holding uncertainty and utilising self-reflectiveness and humility. It is not about being all knowing but being able to stay with the unknown and facilitate the processes of learning from and through experience.

The practice of supervision has developed a framework of theory about supervision, the supervisory relationship and the roles and tasks of a supervisor, but this cannot be prescriptive because with every supervisee and every patient something new enters into the supervisory relationship. As a result, a supervisor needs to be constantly open to and curious about the input and dynamics of the supervisory relationship and begin a process of discovery with their supervisee. Becoming and being a supervisor is an ongoing process and requires an openness to discovery and learning about the supervisory relationship and the processes of supervision. Szecsödy (2014), who has researched and written extensively about supervision, comments that the supervisory process involves 'new learning and relearning' (p.527) and that we should 'never ever stop learning more about supervision' (p.523).

Note

1 My insertions in italics

References

Ekstein, R. and Wallerstein, R.S. (1958) *The Teaching and Learning of Psychotherapy.* Madison Connecticut: International Universities Press, Inc.

Gee, H. (1996) 'Developing insight through supervision. Relating, then defining'. *J. Anal. Psychol.* (41)(4):529–552.

Mander, G. (2002) 'Supervision of supervision: Specialism of new profession?' Driver, C. and Martin, E. (eds.) *Supervising Psychotherapy.* London: Sage Publications.

Power, A. (2013) 'Supervision of supervision: How many mirrors do we need?' *Brit. J. Psychother.* (29)(3):389–404.

Roth, A.D. and Pilling, S. (2015) *A competence framework for the supervision of psychological therapies.* Research Department of Clinical, Educational and Health Psychology. University College London. https://www.ucl.ac.uk/pals/sites/pals/files/background_document_supervision_competences_july_2015.pdf (Accessed 23. 03. 2024).

Szecsödy, I. (2014) 'Prologue: Never ever stop learning more about supervision'. *Psychoanal. Inq.* (34)(6):523–527.

Watkins, C.E. (2014) 'The competent psychoanalytic supervisor: Some thoughts about supervision competences for accountable practice and training'. *Int. Forum Psychoanal.* (23)(4):220–228.

Zachrisson, A. (2011) 'Dynamics of psychoanalytic supervision: A heuristic model'. *Int. J. Psychoanal.* (92)(4):943–961.

Index

For Product Safety Concerns and Information please contact our EU
representative GPSR@taylorandfrancis.com
Taylor & Francis Verlag GmbH, Kaufingerstraße 24, 80331 München, Germany

www.ingramcontent.com/pod-product-compliance
Lightning Source LLC
Chambersburg PA
CBHW071747270326
41928CB00013B/2823